PALEO MONDAY TO FRIDAY

A DIET SO GOOD YOU CAN TAKE THE WEEKEND OFF!

DANIEL GREEN

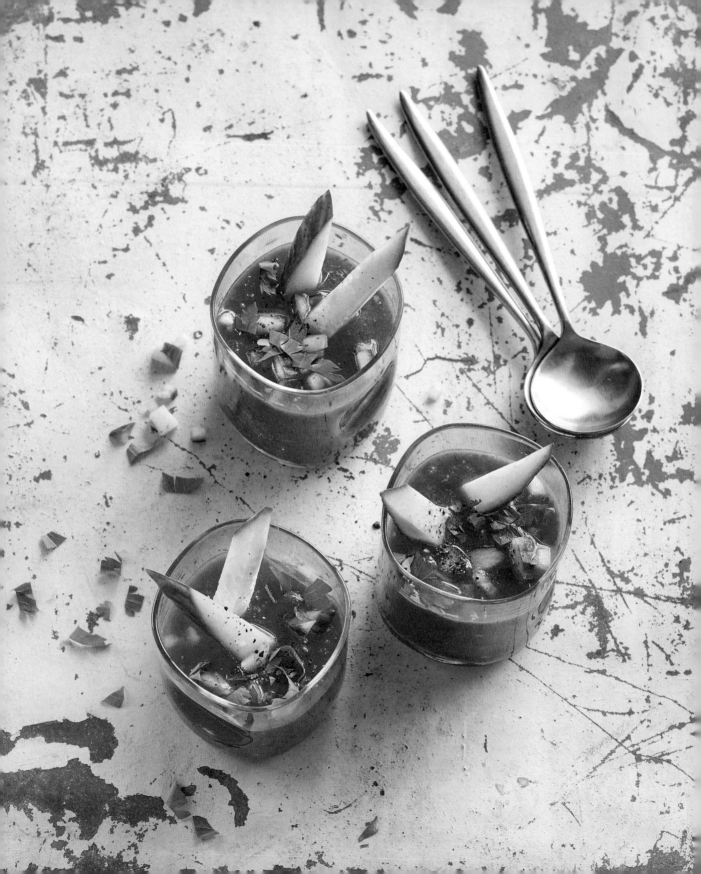

PALEO MONDAY TO FRIDAY

A DIET SO GOOD YOU CAN TAKE THE WEEKEND OFF!

DANIEL GREEN

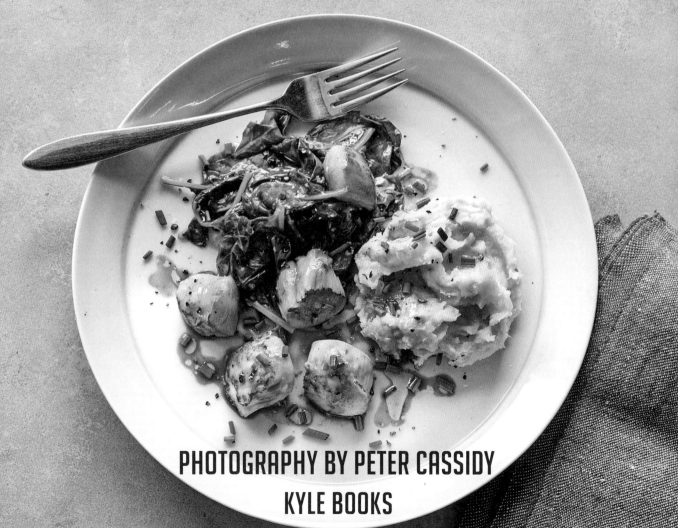

PHOTOGRAPHY BY PETER CASSIDY

KYLE BOOKS

To Georgina with love.
You are a true blessing to our lives.

Published in 2015 by Kyle Books
www.kylebooks.com

Distributed by National Book Network
4501 Forbes Blvd, Suite 200,
Lanham, MD 20706
Phone: (800) 462-6420
Fax: (800) 338-4550
customercare@nbnbooks.com

ISBN: 978 1 909487 44 4

Library of Congress Control Number: 2015960074

Text © Daniel Green 2016
Recipe photographs © Peter Cassidy 2016
Design © Kyle Books 2016

Editor: Vicki Murrell
Design: Anita Mangan
Recipe photography: Peter Cassidy
Food styling: Lizzie Harris
Prop styling: Iris Bromet
Production: Nic Jones and Gemma John

Color reproduction by ALTA London
Printed and bound in China by 1010 Printing International Ltd.

Important notes

All recipe analysis is per portion.

The information and advice contained in this book are intended as a general guide to dieting and healthy eating and are not specific to individuals or their particular circumstances. This book is not intended to replace treatment by a qualified practitioner. Neither the authors nor the publishers can be held responsible for claims arising from the inappropriate use of any dietary regime. Do not attempt self-diagnosis or self-treatment for serious or long-term conditions without consulting a medical professional or qualified practitioner.

The oven temperatures listed in this book are for fan-assisted or convection ovens. If you have a standard oven, simply increase the temperature by about 35 degrees to achieve the same results.

CONTENTS

WHY I LOVE PALEO

In the two years since I published my last book, *The Paleo Diet*, eating Paleo has gone mainstream. To me, its popularity is hardly surprising as the simple principle of cutting out all the synthetic, heavily processed foods that are the cause of our 21st-century bad health and replacing them with the fresh meat, fish, nuts, seeds, fruit, and vegetables that our Paleolithic ancestors thrived on, gives us a food plan that is perfectly suited to our bodies. There is no weighing food, or counting calories. You eat until you are full. There is no starvation or hunger, just satisfying food that tastes great, and as a result, we're healthier and therefore happier.

And if all this sounds good, it gets even better as Paleo also operates according to an "80-20" rule, which means that if 80 percent of what you eat is Paleo, the remaining 20 percent can fall outside. I love this concept, and not because I want an excuse to eat pizza and ice cream and chocolate on my days off, but because it's what makes this diet realistic. It's what I have done for more than 25 years now, since I lost 65 pounds as an overweight young adult, and why over all this time, I've never put the weight back on. I've always followed the exact same rule, which is easy for us to live on and maintain. It's what we do on average that works, and it's why detox diets are so criticized. Why do we expect one detox week out of 52 to make any difference to our health or our weight? It makes sense that it's what we do most of the time that counts. So you love chocolate? Great, you can have it, just in moderation. It's when we deny ourselves things that the cravings build and build and lead to excessive, unhealthy binges and the vicious cycle of yo-yo weight loss and weight gain. It's such a relief that Paleo offers a much healthier and practical alternative!

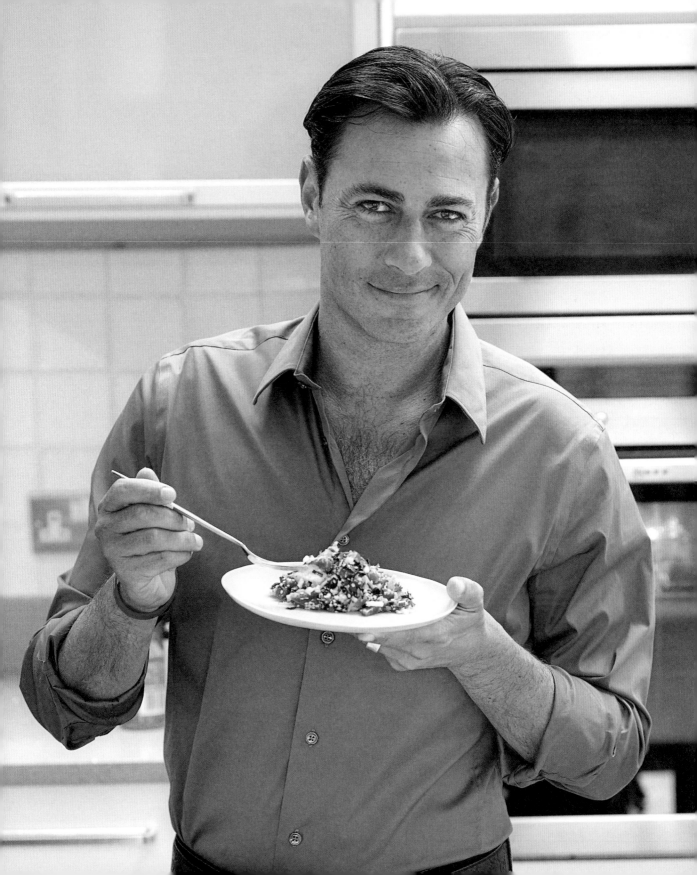

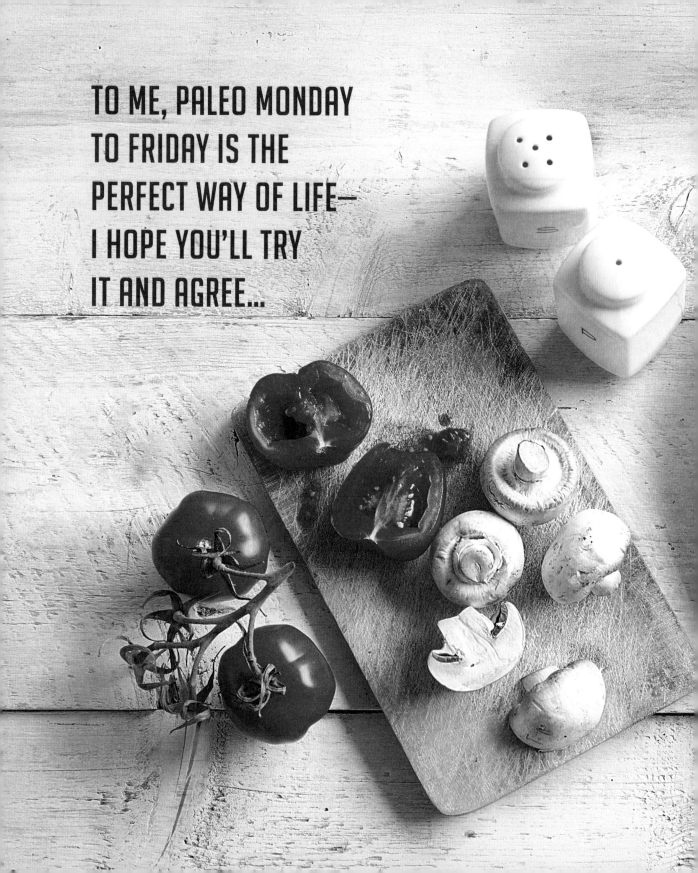

TO ME, PALEO MONDAY
TO FRIDAY IS THE
PERFECT WAY OF LIFE—
I HOPE YOU'LL TRY
IT AND AGREE...

There are some people who don't like the 80-20 rule as they think it provides too much of an opportunity for backsliding and, of course, it's up to you. Also, if you're dealing with serious health problems or intolerances like autoimmune disease, leaky gut, arthritis, and skin rashes, it makes sense to maintain a strict Paleo diet that hopefully eliminates a lot of your symptoms. However, if you are fundamentally healthy, there is no reason why you shouldn't eat a bit of dairy or a few grains or a baked potato now and again. The reality is that we're not living hunter-gatherer lifestyles! We do have times when our routines are disrupted, or we go on holiday or meet friends for dinner, and I love that Paleo acknowledges that there is sometimes more to life than food and escapes the rigid mindset that dooms almost every other diet to fail.

MONDAY TO FRIDAY

So, if you take the 80-20 Paleo rule and apply it to the week, it basically means that if you make good choices from Monday to Friday, you can relax the rules on the weekends. And so this book is all about helping you do just that. I've included recipes for breakfasts, smoothies, snacks, light meals, main meals, and desserts that are simple and easy to prepare during a busy working week. Anyone can make them and the ingredients can be found anywhere. There's loads of variety, as I've picked my favorites from all over the globe, and they're all so delicious and full of flavor that you'll hardly notice you're on a diet. In fact, I don't think of it as one at all. To me, Paleo Monday to Friday is the perfect way of life—I hope you'll try it and agree...

10 REASONS TO EAT THE PALEO WAY

1. It's based on unprocessed, whole foods—which means fewer additives, unhealthy trans fats and no hidden sugars or salt.

2. It's low in salt and rich in potassium—which means lower blood pressure.

3. It's high in fruit and vegetables—which means getting your five servings a day is a cinch.

4. It's low in saturated fat and high in healthy fats—which means lower cholesterol and less inflammation.

5. It's rich in protein and fiber—which means it helps you feel fuller for longer and keeps hunger pangs at bay.

6. It helps to recalibrate your metabolism—which will help you to shed any unwanted weight.

7. It's gluten-free—which helps to banish bloating and digestive problems.

8. It's low GI—which helps to avoid unhealthy spikes in blood sugar.

9. It's rich in plant-based phytochemicals—which can help reduce the risk of certain types of cancer and conditions like dementia.

10. It helps balance the pH in your body—modern diets encourage the production of acid within the body, which is believed to increase calcium loss from the bone and lead to many other health problems, including kidney stones, arthritis, fatigue, headaches, PMS, and skin disorders. In contrast, the Paleo diet helps create a more alkaline environment.

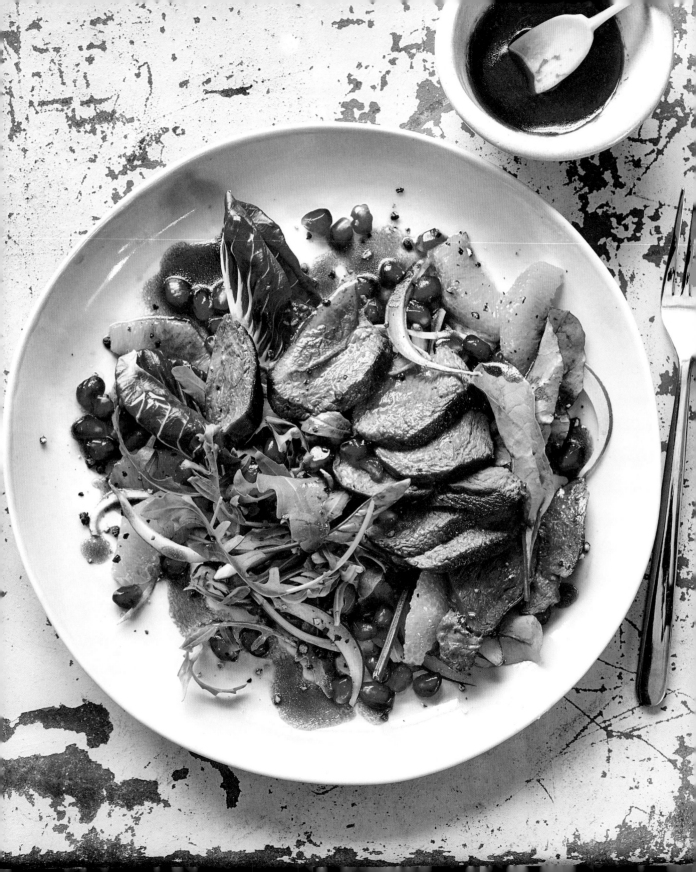

YES

Pile all these good things into your shopping cart and you'll be guaranteed a perfect Paleo diet.

MEAT, FISH & EGGS

eggs—chicken, quail, duck, or even emu.

fish—don't forget fish eggs or roe, which are full of protein and essential vitamins.

FRUIT & VEG

canned fruit and vegetables—check the label to make sure it is sugar- and sodium-free.

NUTS

nut flours—a great ingredient for baking; can be used in place of wheat flour.

nut milks—a great milk substitute. Always choose the unsweetened option, or better still, make your own.

*NB peanuts—don't forget that peanuts are not Paleo-friendly because they are legumes, not nuts.

FLAVORINGS & SAUCES

arrowroot powder—use to thicken sauces in place of cornstarch or wheat flour.

coconut aminos—a soy-free seasoning sauce made from coconut tree sap, this is a great substitute for soy sauce.

curry pastes—make sure you read the label to check the ingredients. It's also very easy to make yourself.

fish sauce—if it has added fructose and sugar or hydrolized wheat protein it is not Paleo. The Red Boat brand is only made from two ingredients (freshly caught wild black anchovies and sea salt) and is minimally processed.

meat, fish and vegetable stocks—organic and low-salt are the best options, or it's very simple to make your own.

mustard—make sure it is gluten- and dairy-free.

salt—sea salt is made through evaporation of ocean water or lake seawater and so undergoes little processing. Table salt is usually mined and contains additives.

tomato purée—make sure it is gluten-free with no added sugar or salts.

SWEETENERS

maple syrup—simply made from the sap of maple trees, this is a lovely, relatively unprocessed natural sweetener.

raw honey—raw, cold-extracted honey hasn't been heat-treated or purified so contains beneficial enzymes and antioxidants.

stevia—a plant that has been used as a sweetener for centuries in Paraguay and Brazil (now commonly available as a naturally sourced sugar substitute).

COCONUT

coconut aminos—see above

coconut flour—also a great substitute for wheat flour.

coconut milk—a great substitute for milk. Look for brands that don't contain guar gum or preservatives.

DRINKS

E.g., filtered or spring water, herbal tea, coconut water, freshly juiced fruit and vegetables

FRUIT & VEG

E.g., apricots, bananas, berries, cherries, citrus fruits, cranberries, dates, dragon fruit, figs, kiwis, lychees, mangos, melons, nectarines, passion fruit, peaches, pears, persimmons, plums, pomegranates, star fruit, artichokes, asparagus, eggplants, broccoli, cabbages, carrots, cauliflowers, zucchini, cucumbers, kale, kohlrabi, leeks, lettuces, okra, olives, onions, bok choy, parsnips, radishes, spinach, watercress, tomatoes, turnips, sea vegetables (kombu, nori, wakame), other seaweeds and algaes, canned fruit and vegetables

SEEDS

E.g., flaxseed, pumpkin seeds, sesame seeds, sunflower seeds

YES

COCONUT

E.g., coconut flour, coconut milk, shredded unsweetened coconut, coconut aminos

OILS & FATS

E.g., avocado oil, coconut oil, flaxseed oil, hazelnut oil, macadamia nut oil, olive oil, sesame oil, walnut oil, lard, tallow

MEAT, FISH & EGGS

E.g., fresh meat, poultry, game and offal, fish and shellfish, eggs

SWEETENERS

E.g., raw honey, stevia, maple syrup

NUTS

E.g., almonds, Brazil nuts, cashews, chestnuts, hazelnuts, macadamias, pecans, pine nuts, pistachios, walnuts, almond flour, almond milk

FLAVORINGS & SAUCES

E.g., fish sauce, curry paste, sea salt, truffle salt, coconut aminos, mustard, tomato purée, stocks, arrowroot powder, herbs and spices

NO

PROCESSED FOODS

WHY? Pumped full of additives, salt, and sugar, the problem is not just with what has been added, but what has been taken away. Processed foods are often stripped of the very nutrient's dietary fibers, vitamins, minerals, and phytochemicals that are good for you.

REFINED & ADDED SUGARS

WHY? Unlike natural sugars (i.e. those you find in fruit, which come packaged with other nutrients), refined sugar provides nothing beneficial. All types of sugar (even unrefined natural sugars like honey) encourage the production of insulin which leads to the laying down of fat.

GRAINS & FOODS CONTAINING GRAINS

WHY? Grains weren't introduced into our diet until after the Agrarian Revolution, so they weren't eaten by our Paleolithic ancestors. Gluten, a protein found in grains, can irritate and damage the lining of the small intestine. This can lead to digestive problems and interfere with the absorption of nutrients from food. Furthermore, in a processed form, grains have a high GI, which means they encourage the release of insulin, which in turn triggers fat storage. They also contain phytic acid, an antinutrient that can block the absorption of important minerals.

BEANS & LEGUMES

WHY? Like cereals, beans and legumes contain antinutrients—lectins and phytic acid—which can irritate and damage the lining of the gut and cause problems such as bloating and diarrhea. The damage caused by lectins is also thought to create a "leaky gut", meaning that other large particles can cross the intestinal barrier and enter your blood stream. This is how food sensitivities start.

VEGETABLE & SEED OILS

WHY? These oils are high in omega-6 fatty acids (very different from heart-healthy omega-3s) and promote inflammation—one of the major causes of heart disease and other conditions such as arthritis.

POTATOES

WHY? Potatoes contain saponins—antinutrients that can damage the intestine. Also, they often have a high glycemic index (GI) value, which means they cause a spike in blood sugar levels that triggers the release of insulin.

DAIRY & FOODS CONTAINING DAIRY

WHY? Cow's milk is designed to help calves grow quickly, not for humans to consume throughout their lives, and many believe we lack the digestive enzymes suited to this task. In fact, humans are the only species to continue drinking milk past weaning and adults in most parts of the world do not consume many dairy products. Some estimates suggest that as much as three-quarters of the world is lactose-intolerant, to varying degrees, with symptoms including gas, bloating, cramps, indigestion, nausea, diarrhea, and constipation.

REFINED & ADDED SUGARS

E.g., sugar, fructose, high fructose corn syrup, corn sugar, corn syrup, agave nectar, golden syrup, malt syrup, molasses, rice syrup, jam, marmalade, jelly, ketchup, hoisin sauce, BBQ sauce

BEANS & LEGUMES

E.g., adzuki beans, baked beans, bean sprouts, black beans, black-eyed peas, broad beans, cannellini beans, chickpeas, kidney beans, lentils, lima beans, mung beans, peas, peanuts, peanut butter, pinto beans, snow peas, sugar snap peas, soy and related products (tofu, miso, soy milk, and soy sauce)

NO

PROCESSED FOODS

E.g., TV dinners, fast food

DAIRY & FOODS CONTAINING DAIRY

E.g., milk, butter, cheese, crème fraîche, cream, ice cream, yogurt

GRAINS & FOODS CONTAINING GRAINS

E.g., flour, barley, rice, corn, sorghum, amaranth, wild rice, buckwheat, spelt, rye, quinoa, bread, pasta, cookies, biscuits, crackers, cakes, bagels, muffins, pancakes, tortilla, couscous, oats, cereal, beer

POTATOES

VEGETABLE & SEED OILS

E.g., rapeseed oil, palm oil, peanut oil, safflower oil, sunflower oil, soy bean oil, margarine

IN MODERATION

ALCOHOL

WHY? The occasional glass of wine isn't a problem and yet it is important to remember that alcohol is a toxin so "in moderation" is key. You should also avoid alcohol that is made from foods on the "avoid" list, such as beer (made from grain), gin (processed with grain-based alcohol), rum (made from sugar), sake (made from rice), vodka (made from potatoes) and whisky (made from grain).

CHOCOLATE

WHY? Chocolate is made from cacao which is packed with healthy chemicals like flavonoids and theobromine. However, chocolate often also contains large amounts of sugar, so ensure you choose a quality brand with a high ratio of cacao solids (i.e. dark rather than milk).

COFFEE

WHY? Coffee can decrease insulin sensitivity, irritate the gastrointestinal tract, and hinder iron absorption. However, it is also full of antioxidants and can protect the liver, so the occasional cup will do no harm. Opt for a quality organic brand as coffee beans are often sprayed with pesticides and other toxins, and don't add sugar!

SALT

WHY? A high-sodium diet will increase the risk of high blood pressure and upset the acid/alkaline balance within the body. I have specifically designed the recipes in this book without much salt and have used other flavorings so that you won't miss it.

STARCHY VEG

WHY? The issue of starchy vegetables is one of Paleo's gray areas. Potatoes are definitely on the "avoid" list, but other root vegetables, such as sweet potatoes, don't contain the same antinutrients and don't have such an adverse effect on blood sugar levels. Many hunter-gatherer groups, such as the Kitavans of Papua New Guinea, regularly eat yams, sweet potatoes, taro, and cassava (tapioca), and don't suffer any adverse effects. For this reason I include them here in the "in moderation" group.

SWEETENERS

WHY? The body processes all forms of sugar in the same way (even honey produces an insulin response in the body), so I recommend you only use raw honey, maple syrup or stevia (in moderation) as sweeteners. Raw honey is honey in its purest, most unprocessed form (it still contains many of the nutrients that the bees put into it). Stevia is a natural, plant-sourced, calorie-free sugar substitute.

VINEGAR

WHY? Strictly speaking, vinegar wasn't introduced to the human diet until after the Agrarian Revolution, so it wasn't around in Paleolithic times—if you do want to use vinegar in moderation, choose apple cider vinegar, balsamic or red/white wine vinegar rather than barley malt vinegar. Vinegar can upset the acid/alkaline balance within the body, so use it only in moderation.

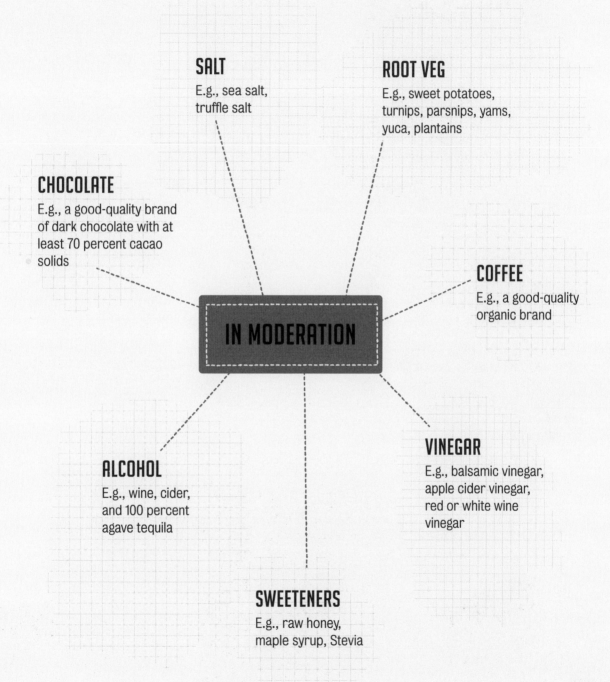

SALT
E.g., sea salt, truffle salt

ROOT VEG
E.g., sweet potatoes, turnips, parsnips, yams, yuca, plantains

CHOCOLATE
E.g., a good-quality brand of dark chocolate with at least 70 percent cacao solids

COFFEE
E.g., a good-quality organic brand

IN MODERATION

ALCOHOL
E.g., wine, cider, and 100 percent agave tequila

VINEGAR
E.g., balsamic vinegar, apple cider vinegar, red or white wine vinegar

SWEETENERS
E.g., raw honey, maple syrup, Stevia

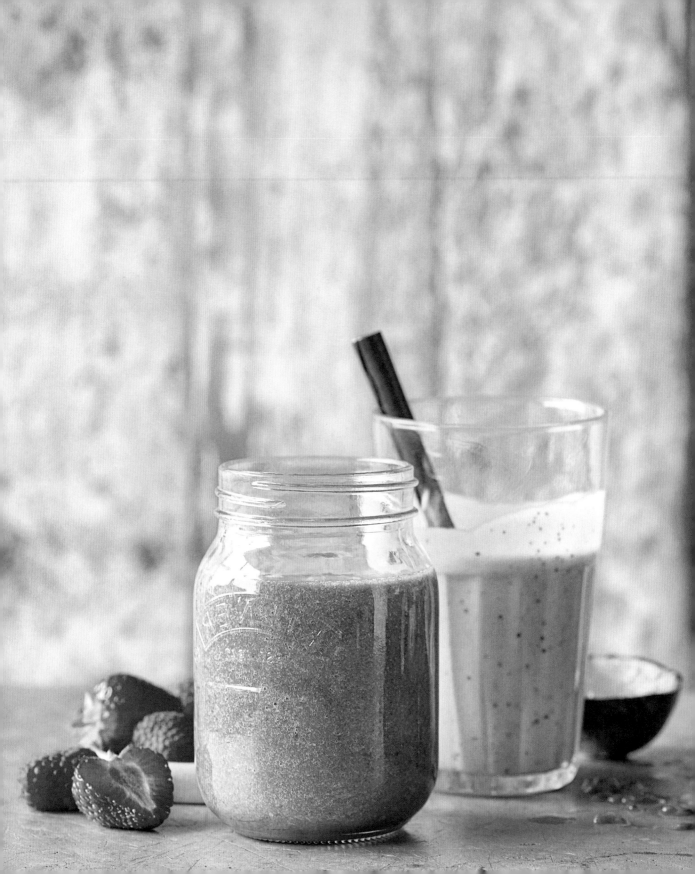

BREAKFASTS
& BRUNCHES

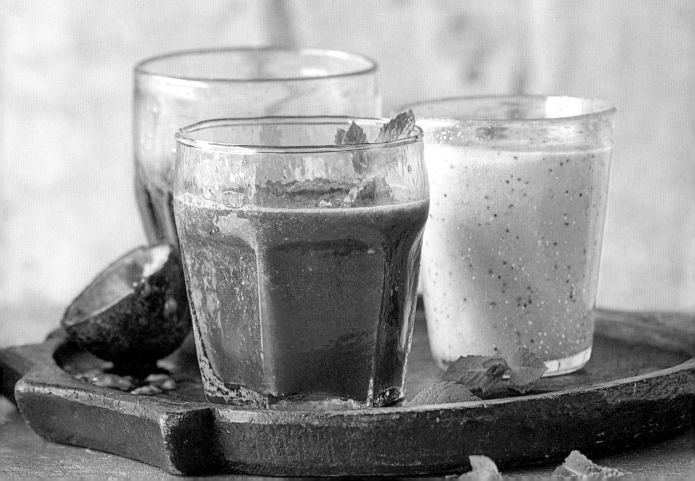

SUN-DRIED TOMATO OMELET
WITH MEXICAN SALSA

When I spent time in Mexico, I discovered how salsas are such a great accompaniment to eggs. They're so fresh and spicy and make a fantastic breakfast or brunch, especially in the summer.

340 CALORIES | 23G FAT | 4.5G SATURATES | 11.5G CARBS | 11G SUGAR | 1.1G SALT | 21G PROTEIN | 3.5G FIBER

- -

SERVES 2

for the salsa

4 plum tomatoes, seeded and finely chopped

6 fresh basil leaves, finely chopped

a handful of fresh cilantro leaves, finely chopped

¼ yellow onion, finely chopped

juice of ½ lime

1 small jalapeño pepper, finely chopped

4 eggs

2 egg whites

sea salt and freshly ground black pepper

olive oil spray, for frying

¾ cup sun-dried tomatoes in olive oil, drained and finely sliced

2 scallions, sliced

1. First make the salsa: Place all the ingredients in a large bowl and mix together well.

2. Break the eggs into a separate bowl, lightly season, and beat together with a fork.

3. Place a frying pan over high heat, spray with a little olive oil and add the eggs, tilting the pan to spread the mixture evenly over the base, then lower the heat to medium. After a minute or two, use a spatula to pull the outer edges of the omelet into the center. The liquid, uncooked egg will fill the space and ensure the omelet cooks evenly and the base doesn't burn.

4. When almost all the egg is cooked, add the sun-dried tomatoes, then use a spatula again to flip one side of the omelet over so it is folded in half.

5. Take off the heat, rest for 30 seconds, and then serve immediately with the chopped scallions sprinkled on top and the salsa on the side.

- -

TIP You can make this the night before as it keeps well in the refrigerator. Take the chile seeds out if you don't want too much of a kick too early in the morning!

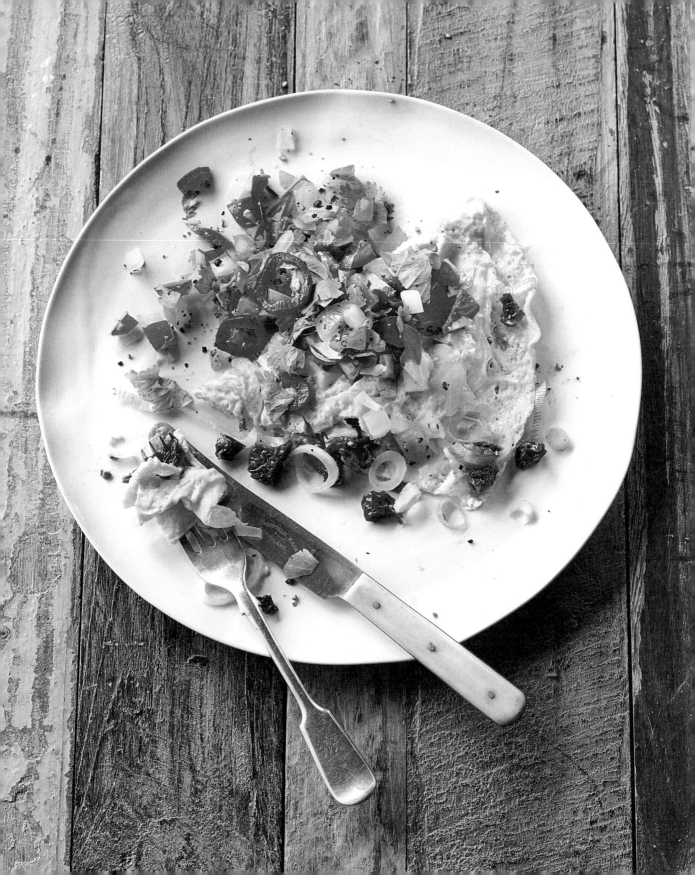

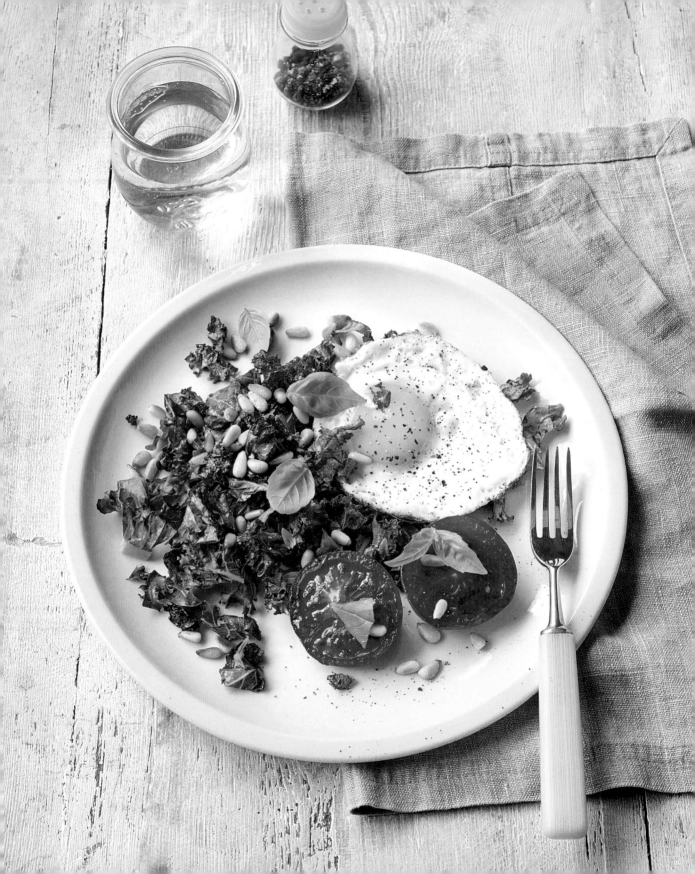

KALE & EGGS
WITH GRIDDLED TOMATOES

Kale is very close to spinach in nutritional values (loaded with vitamins, minerals, antioxidants, and phytonutrients) but it has a little more texture and strength so it holds its shape when you cook with it. Also, its bulk means it's filling and sets you up for the day, which makes it perfect for breakfast.

467 CALORIES | 34.5G FAT | 7G SATURATES | 7G CARBS | 7G SUGAR | 0.8G SALT | 28.5G PROTEIN | 6.5G FIBER

SERVES 2

1 tablespoon pine nuts

2 tablespoons olive oil

4 large tomatoes, thickly sliced

7 ounces (about 3 cups) kale leaves, stemmed

6 to 8 fresh basil leaves, shredded

6 eggs

1. Place a large non-stick frying pan over medium to high heat and, when hot, toast the pine nuts (with no oil) until they turn brown this will only take a minute or two. Transfer the pine nuts to a dish and set aside.

2. Add a drizzle of oil to the same pan and fry the tomatoes for about 2 minutes on each side. Again, transfer to a dish and set aside.

3. Now turn up the heat, add a tablespoon of oil to the pan and stir-fry the kale for a few minutes until it chars and turns a little crispy. Add the shredded basil and toasted pine nuts to the pan and toss together.

4. Meanwhile, heat the remaining oil in a large frying pan and, when hot, crack in each egg, being careful not to crowd the pan. Cover and leave for a few minutes, then check the white is cooked, lift out and transfer to a plate.

5. Serve the eggs immediately with the griddled tomatoes and kale, and garnish with a little fresh basil.

TIP This recipe serves up 3 eggs per person. It may seem like a lot, but scientific research has debunked the myth that dietary cholesterol causes heart disease and actually proves that eating up to 3 whole eggs per day is a great way for a healthy person to stay healthy. Enjoy!

EGG & EGG WHITE OMELET

Eggs are high in dietary cholesterol (185mg per egg) and this is all contained in the egg's yolk, so back when scientists thought that dietary cholesterol was linked to blood cholesterol and heart disease, egg yolks started to get a bad name. This is a shame as the yolk is in fact a powerhouse of nutrition and the fat it contains even helps to reduce LDL (bad cholesterol) in the blood. However, as many of the breakfast recipes in this book contain many eggs, I've made an omelet here with a 2:1 ratio of egg white to egg yolk as, for me, it still has the perfect golden color and creamy texture, but tastes a little less rich.

155 CALORIES | 10G FAT | 2.5G SATURATES | 0G CARBS | 0G SUGAR | 0.6G SALT | 17G PROTEIN | 0G FIBER

- -

SERVES 2

3 eggs

3 egg whites

sea salt and freshly ground
   black pepper

1 teaspoon olive oil

your choice of fillings
   (see below)

1. Break the eggs into a bowl, lightly season, and beat together with a fork.

2. Place a frying pan over high heat and add the olive oil, then fry the filling ingredients of your choice (see below) for a minute or two until cooked.

3. Add the eggs, tilting the pan to spread the mixture evenly over the base, then lower the heat to medium. After a minute or two, use a spatula to pull the outer edges of the omelet into the center. The uncooked egg will fill the space and ensure the omelet cooks evenly and the base doesn't burn.

4. When almost all the egg is cooked, use a spatula again to flip one side of the omelet over so it is folded in half. Take off the heat, rest for 30 seconds, then serve immediately.

- -

TIP All these ingredients taste delicious finely chopped in an omelet. I recommend using whatever meat and vegetables you have in your refrigerator at the time as a way of keeping the flavors and combinations nice and varied: sun-dried tomatoes, onions, mushrooms, peppers, tomatoes, ham, chicken, turkey, lean bacon, chives, flat-leaf parsley.

RED ONION & SPINACH OMELET

Eggs are among the most nutritious foods on the planet and spinach is a superfood loaded with health benefits (full of iron, vitamins, and minerals) so this omelet makes a breakfast of champions.

181 CALORIES | 10G FAT | 2.5G SATURATES | 2G CARBS | 1.5G SUGAR | 0.7G SALT | 20G PROTEIN | 1.1G FIBER

SERVES 2

1 teaspoon olive oil

¼ red onion, finely chopped

3½ ounces (about 2½ cups) fresh spinach

3 eggs

4 egg whites

sea salt and freshly ground black pepper

1. Place the olive oil in a non-stick frying pan over high heat. Add the onion and fry for a minute, then add the spinach and cook until wilted. Transfer to a plate and set aside.

2. Crack the eggs into a bowl, season lightly and beat with a fork.

3. Now make one omelet at a time: Tip half the egg mixture into the hot pan, tilting to spread the mixture evenly over the base, then distribute half the cooked onion and spinach on top.

4. After a minute or two, use a spatula to pull the outer edges of the omelet into the centre. The uncooked egg will fill the space and ensure the omelet cooks evenly and the base doesn't burn.

5. When almost all the egg is cooked, use a spatula again to flip one side of the omelet over so it is folded in half.

6. Take off the heat, rest for 30 seconds, then serve immediately. Repeat steps 3 to 5 for the second omelet.

TIP The omelet will continue to cook after you have taken it off the heat so don't overcook it in the pan and don't rest it for too long either. Serve while it is still nice and hot.

PORK PATTIES
WITH HOMEMADE TOMATO KETCHUP

This dish is a great alternative to a traditional meaty cooked breakfast and also makes a great lunch or dinner, served with a nice fresh salad.

274 CALORIES | 10G FAT | 4G SATURATES | 12G CARBS | 10G SUGAR | 0.3G SALT | 33G PROTEIN | 1.5G FIBER

SERVES 4

olive oil spray, for frying

a handful of flat-leaf parsley, to garnish

for the tomato ketchup

1 × 14.5-ounce can puréed tomatoes

6 tablespoons tomato paste

¼ cup white vinegar

1½ tablespoons maple syrup

for the patties

1 pound lean ground pork

1 egg

1 teaspoon ground cumin

1 teaspoon red pepper flakes

1 tablespoon chopped fresh parsley

1 small yellow onion, finely chopped

1 garlic clove, crushed

2 tablespoons homemade tomato ketchup (see above)

1. First make the tomato ketchup: Place all the ingredients in a saucepan and stir to combine. Bring to a boil over medium heat, then turn down to a simmer, cover, turn off the heat, and let stand for 5 minutes.

2. Meanwhile, make the patties: Place all the ingredients in a large bowl and use your hands to mix together well. When thoroughly combined, shape the mince into 2-inch patties. You should have enough to make a dozen or so.

3. Place a large frying pan over high heat and lightly spray with oil. When hot, fry the patties for 2 to 3 minutes on each side until cooked through.

4. Stir the tomato ketchup again and serve with the patties, with a little fresh parsley to garnish.

TIP You can buy your own pork and grind it yourself in a food processor. In fact, I recommend doing this whenever you cook with ground meat as then you know exactly how fresh it is and what's in it.

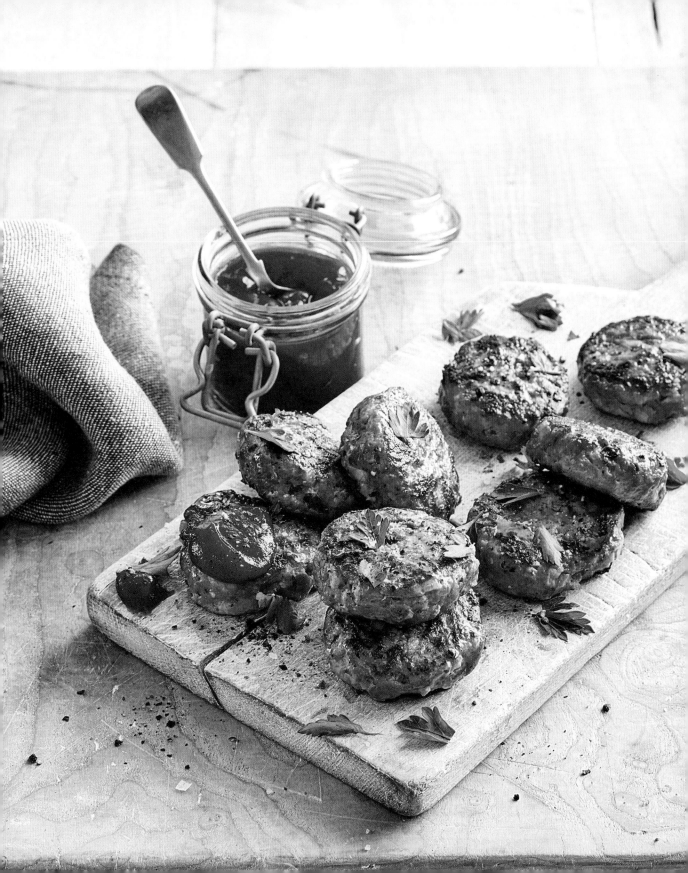

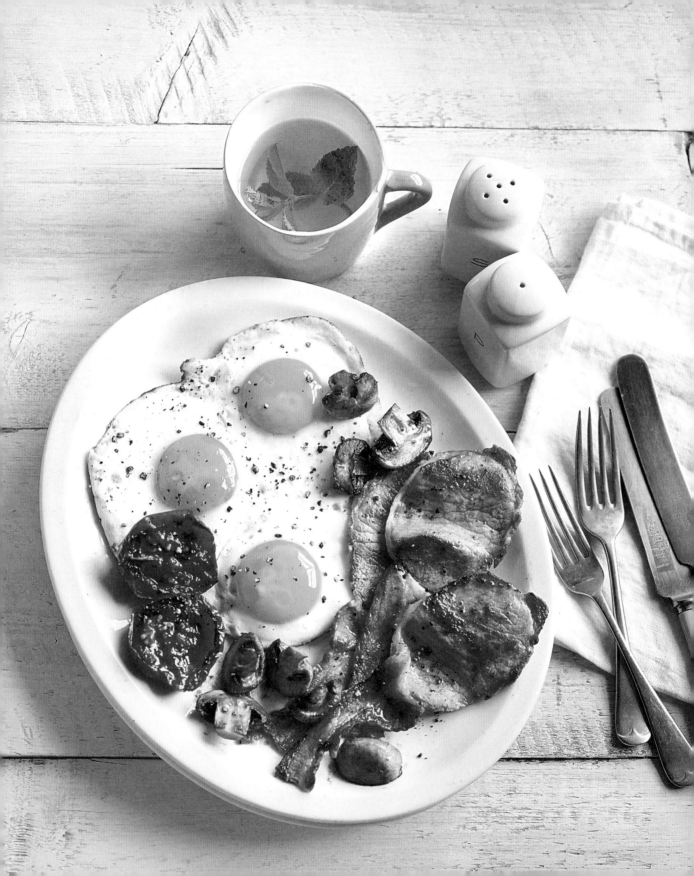

BACON & EGGS

The Full English Breakfast started to get a bad name when fat was demonized back in the 1950s. However, there really is no evidence that high-fat foods lead to heart disease and weight gain. In fact, they fill you up faster (so you'll eat less) and for longer than high-carb foods so forget the toast and the hash browns and you can enjoy this guiltless pleasure.

480 CALORIES | 36G FAT | 11G SATURATES | 3G CARBS | 3G SUGAR | 2.7G SALT | 35G PROTEIN | 1.5G FIBER

- -

SERVES 4

1½ tablespoons olive oil

12 small white mushrooms, cleaned and quartered

3 plum tomatoes, halved

12 slices Canadian bacon, trimmed of fat

12 eggs (3 per person)

freshly ground black pepper

4 sprigs fresh parsley

1. Heat 1 tablespoon olive oil in a large non-stick frying pan and stir-fry the mushrooms for 2 to 3 minutes over high heat. Lower the heat a little, add the tomatoes and cook for another 2 to 3 minutes, turning them halfway through, then transfer to a plate and keep warm.

2. Place the bacon in the same pan and fry over medium heat for a minute or two on each side.

3. Meanwhile, spray another large non-stick frying pan with a little oil and, when hot, crack in each egg, being careful not to crowd the pan. Cover and leave for a few minutes, then check the white is cooked, lift out and transfer to a plate.

4. Serve everything together with a sprinkle of ground pepper and fresh parsley for color.

- -

TIP The best way to clean mushrooms is to wipe them with a paper towel. This doesn't add any moisture and yet still cleans them well.

MUSHROOM & ONION WRAP

The coconut flour gives this pancake a lovely sweet flavor. It can be quite delicate so allow it to sit in the pan and firm up a little before you flip it.

416 CALORIES | 32G FAT | 3G SATURATES | 12.5G CARBS | 5G SUGAR | 0.2G SALT | 15G PROTEIN | 6G FIBER

SERVES 4

olive oil spray, for frying

3½ ounces (about 1½ cups) white mushrooms, roughly chopped

¼ red onion, finely sliced

3 egg whites

4 tablespoons coconut flour

1. Place a large non-stick frying pan over high heat, spray with a little olive oil, and stir-fry the mushrooms for 3 minutes or so until they start to brown. Add the onion and stir-fry for an additional 2 to 3 minutes, then remove from the pan and keep warm.

2. Crack the egg into a small bowl, add the egg white and beat lightly with a fork. Add the coconut flour and stir to combine.

3. Place the clean non-stick pan back on medium heat and spray with a little olive oil. Ladle a quarter of the pancake batter into the pan and swirl to coat the base evenly. Leave to cook for 2 minutes or so. When firm, flip the pancake and cook the other side for 2 minutes. When lightly brown, add a quarter of the onion and mushroom mixture and then fold the pancake over so the filling is sealed inside.

4. Make the remaining pancakes, then simply slide onto a plate, and serve immediately.

TIP Coconut flour is a great Paleo-friendly alternative to wheat flour—it's nutrient-rich, full of fiber, and low GI, which means it supports a healthy metabolism and stable blood sugar levels.

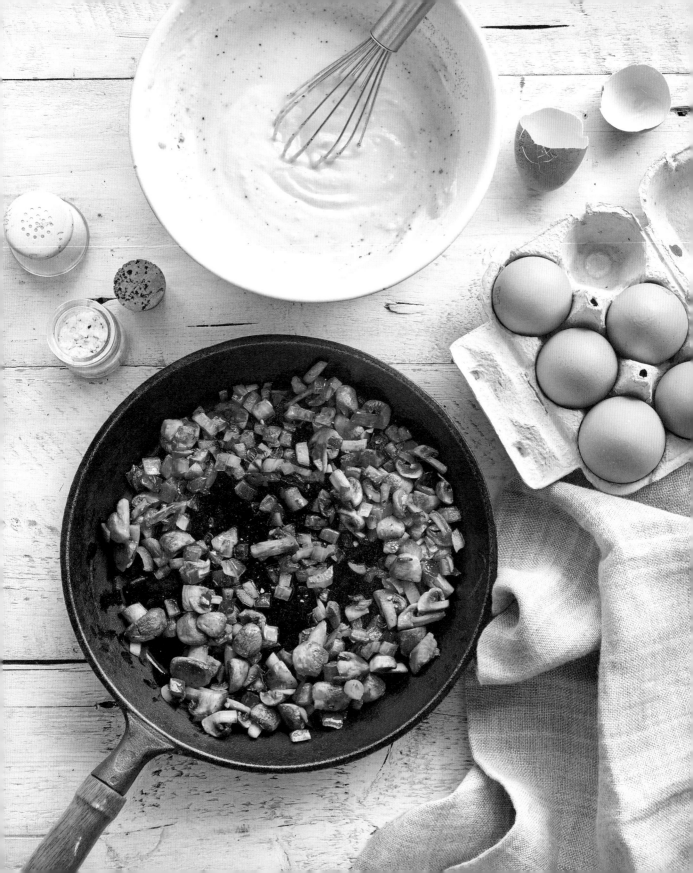

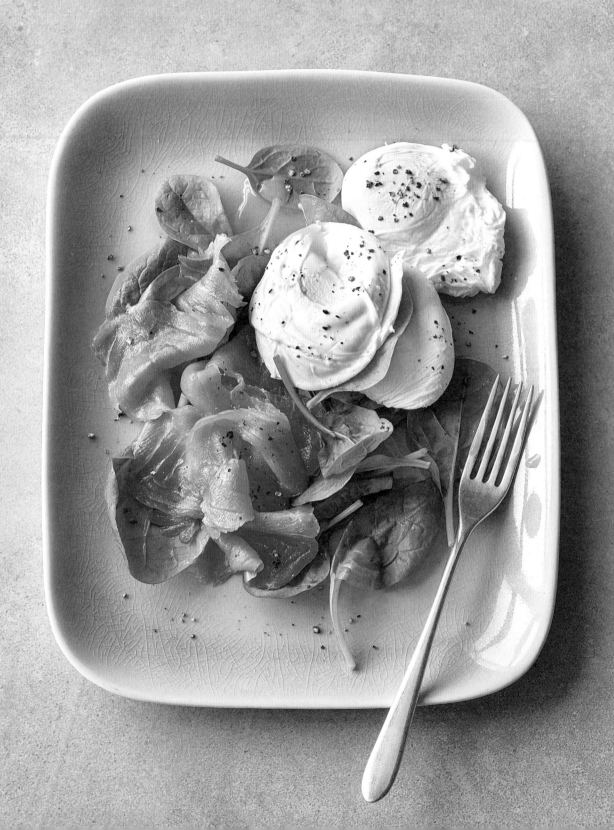

POACHED EGGS
ON SMOKED SALMON & SPINACH

Poaching is probably the very best way to cook eggs—it's so easy and you don't add a single drop of extra fat. However, don't forget to use the freshest eggs you can afford as it'll make all the difference.

617 CALORIES | 38G FAT | 10G SATURATES | 2G CARBS | 2G SUGAR | 7G SALT | 66G PROTEIN | 3G FIBER

SERVES 2

a dash of white vinegar

6 eggs

7 ounces (about 5 cups) fresh spinach

12 ounces Scottish smoked salmon, thinly sliced

Freshly ground black pepper

1. Bring a large saucepan of water to a boil and add a dash of white vinegar. Crack each egg individually into a ramekin or small cup and then slide it into the water. It's important not to overcrowd the pan so I recommend you only cook three at a time. Cook the eggs for a minute at a rolling boil, then reduce to a simmer and cook for an additional 2 minutes.

2. Remove the eggs with a slotted spoon and place briefly in a pan of cold water to remove any trace of vinegar, then place on a paper towel.

3. Place a pile of spinach leaves on each individual plate and top with smoked salmon and three poached eggs. Finish with a twist of black pepper and serve immediately.

TIP Free-range chickens grubbing in a field are far healthier than ones kept in cages and studies have shown their eggs are nutritionally superior.

JAPANESE EGG CUSTARDS

These little steamed egg custards are traditionally served for breakfast in Japan. They're delicious and savory and keep you feeling full right up until lunch. I also like to serve these with finely sliced mushrooms or scallions and you can substitute the salmon for small shrimp if you like.

168 CALORIES | 10G FAT | 2G SATURATES | 1.5G CARBS | 1G SUGAR | 0.8G SALT | 18G PROTEIN | 2G FIBER

SERVES 4

4 eggs

2 egg whites

vegetable stock or dashi (you need equal ratio of stock to egg)

4 ounces (about ½ cup) flaked cooked or canned salmon

4 large broccoli florets, quartered

1. Crack the eggs into a medium-sized bowl and, using chopsticks, lightly whisk until blended, without incorporating too much air. Stir in the dashi or stock (a 50:50 ratio of egg to stock).

2. Divide the flaked salmon between four small serving bowls or ramekins and pour the egg mixture on top. Cover the bowls or wrap them in plastic wrap and steam over low heat (the water should be at a gentle simmer) for 15 to 20 minutes, or until the eggs are set—a bamboo steamer is great for this.

3. Immediately transfer the bowls to the refrigerator to chill for at least 3 hours or overnight.

4. Unwrap the custards. Place the broccoli florets in a bamboo steamer over a pan of gently simmering water and steam for 3 to 4 minutes.

5. Top the custards with the broccoli and serve.

TIP In order to achieve the perfect velvety-smooth texture, cook these little custards on the lowest heat you can manage.

COOKED APPLES IN MAPLE SYRUP
WITH AN ALMOND CRUMB

This is the perfect warming, filling breakfast to eat on a cold winter's morning.
Or it could make a very tasty dessert, too.

544 CALORIES | 29G FAT | 2.5G SATURATES | 52G CARBS | 49G SUGAR | 0G SALT | 13G PROTEIN | 5G FIBER

SERVES 2

4 apples, peeled, cored, and
  roughly chopped
1 teaspoon ground cinnamon
2 tablespoons maple syrup
1 cup ground almonds
a handful of fresh blackberries

1. Preheat the grill to its highest setting.

2. Place the apples in a saucepan with ½ cup of
water, then add the cinnamon and 1 tablespoon
of maple syrup. Bring to a boil, cover, and
simmer for about 7 minutes, then remove the
lid and cook for an additional minute to allow
any excess liquid to evaporate.

3. Divide the cooked apple between four
ovenproof ramekins and cover each one with
almond flour and a drizzle of maple syrup. Place
under the grill for a minute or so, being careful
not to burn.

4. Serve with a few fresh blackberries on the side.

TIP Almond flour has a wonderful texture and flavor, plus
it's very low in carbs, full of magnesium and vitamin
E and monounsaturated fats, and contains a very
healthy amount of protein.

BERRY COMPOTE
WITH A COCONUT CRUST

This breakfast is excellent at filling the gap when you are craving carbs.
I recommend that you make it the night before, then simply place it
under the broiler in the morning.

231 CALORIES | 6G FAT | 4G SATURATES | 28G CARBS | 14G SUGAR | 0.2G SALT | 8G PROTEIN | 15G FIBER

SERVES 4

12 ounces blackberries

6 ounces raspberries

2 tablespoons maple syrup

1 cup coconut flour

1 egg, beaten

Scant ¼ cup unsweetened
  almond milk

1. Turn the broiler to its highest setting.

2. Place the blackberries and raspberries in a
   saucepan with 2 tablespoons water and add
   the maple syrup. Bring to a boil and cook for
   2 to 3 minutes, then turn down the heat and
   simmer for 4 to 5 minutes (so the berries keep
   their shape).

3. Meanwhile, mix the coconut flour with the egg
   and almond milk until it's crumbly and looks
   like streusel.

4. Divide the cooked berries, reserving the juices,
   between four ovenproof ramekins and top with
   the coconut streusel. Drizzle over a little more
   maple syrup and place under the hot broiler for
   3 to 4 minutes, being careful not to let it burn.
   Serve warm with a drizzle of the reserved
   berry juice.

TIP Fresh fruit is great and "fresh is best" is often used as
a healthy eating mantra. However, research has shown
that frozen fruit and veg actually provide the same health
benefits as fresh and can even retain their nutritional value
for longer as they're preserved at their peak. Frozen
berries work perfectly for this recipe as they are cooked
down and therefore don't have to look freshly picked and
beautiful.

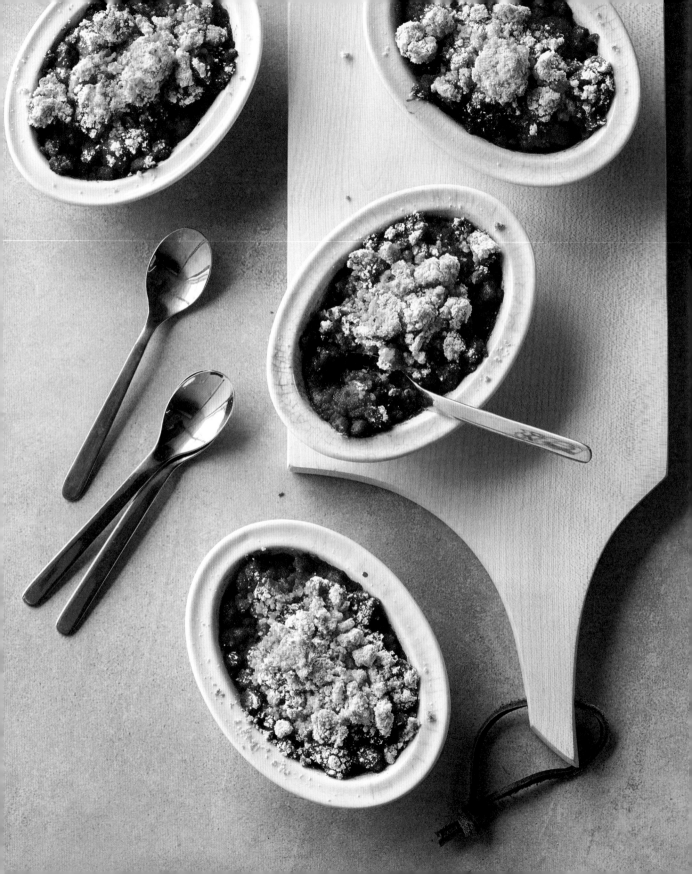

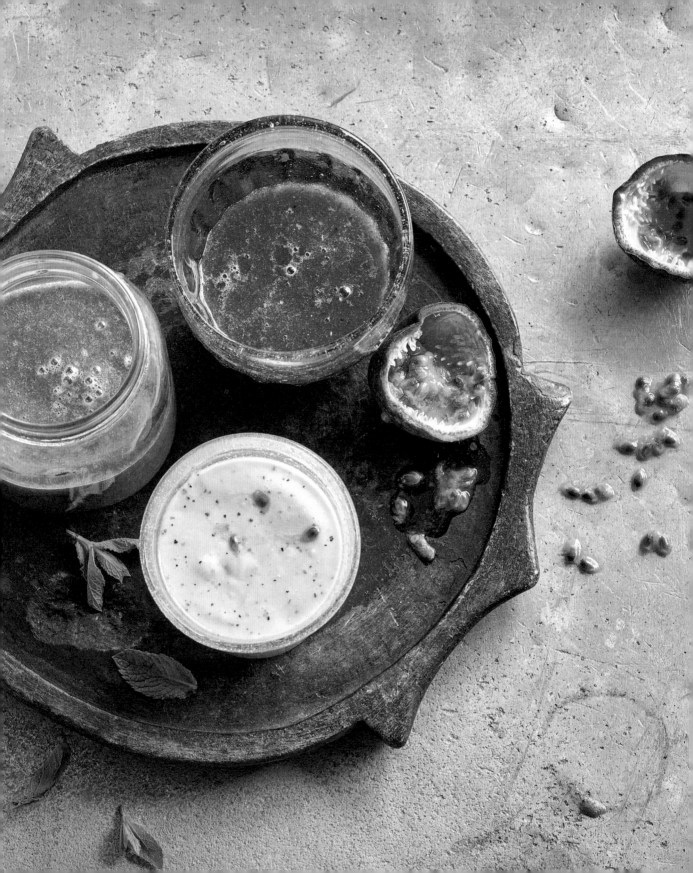

SMOOTHIES

MANGO SMOOTHIE

This makes such a delicious, sweet, and creamy smoothie, and it's perfectly refreshing.

138 CALORIES | 1.5G FAT | 0.5G SATURATES | 26G CARBS | 26G SUGAR | 0.2G SALT | 2G PROTEIN | 5G FIBER

SERVES 2

1 medium mango, peeled and pitted
1 cup unsweetened almond milk
juice of 1 orange
juice of ½ lemon
8 to 10 ice cubes

1. Place all the ingredients in a blender and process until smooth.

2. Pour into glasses and serve immediately.

STRAWBERRY ENERGIZER

I know that coffee is not strictly Paleo but I also know that most people need a caffeine fix now and again. The best advice I think is to save it for those times when you need it most...

64 CALORIES | 2G FAT | 0.2G SATURATES | 9G CARBS | 9G SUGAR | 0.1G SALT | 1G PROTEIN | 4G FIBER

SERVES 2

7 ounces (about 1 cup) fresh strawberries, hulled
1 shot espresso
1 cup unsweetened almond milk
8 to 10 ice cubes

1. Place all the ingredients in a blender and process until smooth.

2. Pour into glasses and serve immediately.

MORNING ENERGIZER

The banana here will provide you with plenty of energy. However, you can also add a little coffee (see Tip below) if it's a day off.

104 CALORIES | 1.5G FAT | 0.2G SATURATES | 20G CARBS | 19G SUGAR | 0.2G SALT | 1.5G PROTEIN | 0.7G FIBER

SERVES 2

1¼ cups unsweetened almond milk

1 tablespoon maple syrup

1 ripe banana

1. Place all the ingredients in a blender and process until smooth.

2. Pour into glasses and serve immediately.

TIP Coffee is a no on strict Paleo, but if it's the weekend and you feel you need a little extra energy, add 1 freshly made espresso shot to the blender before you process.

KALE & BERRY SMOOTHIE

This is a great detox drink. Kale is the top superfood of the moment and with good reason—it's incredibly low in calories and yet amazingly rich in nutrients (especially the minerals many of us are deficient in) and if you simply eat more kale you will significantly improve the total nutrient content in your diet.

123 CALORIES | TRACE FAT | TRACE SATURATES | 22G CARBS | 22G SUGAR | 0G SALT | 3G PROTEIN | 7G FIBER

SERVES 2

¾ cup kale leaves, stemmed

1⅓ cups freshly squeezed orange juice

7 ounces (about 1 cup) strawberries, hulled

3½ ounces (⅔ cup) raspberries

1. Place all the ingredients in a blender and process until smooth.

2. Pour into glasses and serve immediately.

TIP Smoothies taste best when they are freshest. The ingredients can separate and the texture can become thick or gelatinous if they're left to sit and so I always recommend you drink them right away.

ASIAN FRUIT SMOOTHIE WITH PASSION FRUIT

Most fruits from Southeast Asia are deliciously sweet and mango and papaya are no exception. However, as they are so high in sugar (and therefore also high in carbs), use a little sparingly and save for a treat.

132 CALORIES | 3.5G FAT | 2G SATURATES | 20G CARBS | 20G SUGAR | 0.1G SALT | 2G PROTEIN | 5.5G FIBER

SERVES 2

½ small mango, peeled and pitted

½ small papaya, peeled and seeded

⅔ cup unsweetened almond milk

¼ cup light coconut milk

2 passion fruit, halved

1. Place the mango and papaya in a blender with the milks and process until smooth.

2. Pour into glasses, then scoop out the seeds of the passion fruit and float on top of each smoothie. Serve immediately.

FROZEN BERRY SMOOTHIE

Frozen berries are very nutritious as the berries are picked and frozen when they're ripe and in their prime. However, try not to keep them in the freezer for longer than 6 months to a year.

80 CALORIES | 0G FAT | 0G SATURATES | 16G CARBS | 16G SUGAR | 0G SALT | 2G PROTEIN | 3G FIBER

SERVES 2

9 ounces (about 1¾ cups) frozen berries (a mix of raspberries, blackberries, and strawberries are best)

1 cup freshly squeezed orange juice

3 to 4 sprigs fresh mint (optional)

1. Place the berries with the orange juice in a blender and process until smooth. Add a little more juice to thin out the mixture if it becomes a little thick.

2. Pour into glasses and serve with a sprig of mint.

CUCUMBER & MINT DETOX

This is the BEST smoothie ever—fresh, filling, and incredibly tasty. If I were you, I'd try this before any of the others.

123 CALORIES | 8G FAT | 1.5G SATURATES | 8G CARBS | 8G SUGAR | 0G SALT | 3G PROTEIN | 3G FIBER

SERVES 2

¾ cucumber, sliced

2 tablespoons torn fresh mint leaves

juice of 2 oranges (add the flesh if you want a thicker smoothie)

½ ripe avocado, peeled and pitted

4 to 6 ice cubes

1. Place the cucumber, mint, and orange juice in a blender and process until smooth. Add the avocado and process again, adding a little more juice if the mixture becomes a little thick and your blender struggles.

2. Pour into glasses over ice and serve with a garnish of fresh mint.

TIP Cucumbers are great for detoxing as they're diuretics and so help you to avoid water retention and flush toxins out of the body.

WATERMELON & MINT SMOOTHIE

I love this drink as it tastes of summer, even during the darkest winter. Simply increase or decrease the quantity of mint to suit your taste.

54 CALORIES | 0G FAT | 0G SATURATES | 11G CARBS | 11G SUGAR | 0G SALT | 0.8G PROTEIN | 0.2G FIBER

SERVES 2

2 cups watermelon flesh, cut into chunks

2 to 3 tablespoons fresh mint leaves

8 to 10 ice cubes

1. Place the ingredients in a blender and process until smooth.

2. Pour into glasses over ice and serve immediately.

TIP On a weekend, I recommend you serve this over ice and add a shot of Cîroc vodka, which is made from grapes rather than potatoes!

VITAMIN C BLAST

This refreshing drink provides you with more nutrients than any vitamin C pill, plus it boosts your immune system, wards off colds and infections, and tastes delicious.

154 CALORIES | 0G FAT | 0G SATURATES | 30G CARBS | 30G SUGAR | 0G SALT | 3G PROTEIN | 6G FIBER

SERVES 2

3 oranges, peeled and excess pith removed

2 grapefruits, peeled and excess pith removed

juice of 1 lemon

1 tablespoon torn fresh mint leaves

1. Place the orange and grapefruit segments in a blender with the lemon juice and mint and process until smooth.

2. Pour into glasses and serve immediately.

COCONUT MILK & MANGO SMOOTHIE

This smoothie provides a great natural energy boost, plus it's very filling and you won't need anything else for breakfast.

263 CALORIES | 16G FAT | 13G SATURATES | 26G CARBS | 24G SUGAR | 0.1G SALT | 2.5G PROTEIN | 5G FIBER

SERVES 2

¾ cup coconut milk

Scant ½ cup unsweetened almond milk

1 small ripe mango, peeled and pitted

½ banana, peeled

1. Place all the ingredients in a blender and process until smooth.

2. Pour into glasses and serve immediately.

ALMOND BERRY BLAST

I recommend you source the unsweetened version of almond milk if you are watching your weight as the "original" varieties often contain as much as 7 grams of sugar per carton.

117 CALORIES | 2G FAT | 0.2G SATURATES | 18G CARBS | 18G SUGAR | 0.2G SALT | 2.6G PROTEIN | 7G FIBER

SERVES 2

1¼ cups unsweetened almond milk

5 ounces strawberries

3½ ounces raspberries

3½ ounces blackberries

½ ripe banana

1. Place all the ingredients in a blender and process until smooth.

2. Pour into glasses and serve immediately.

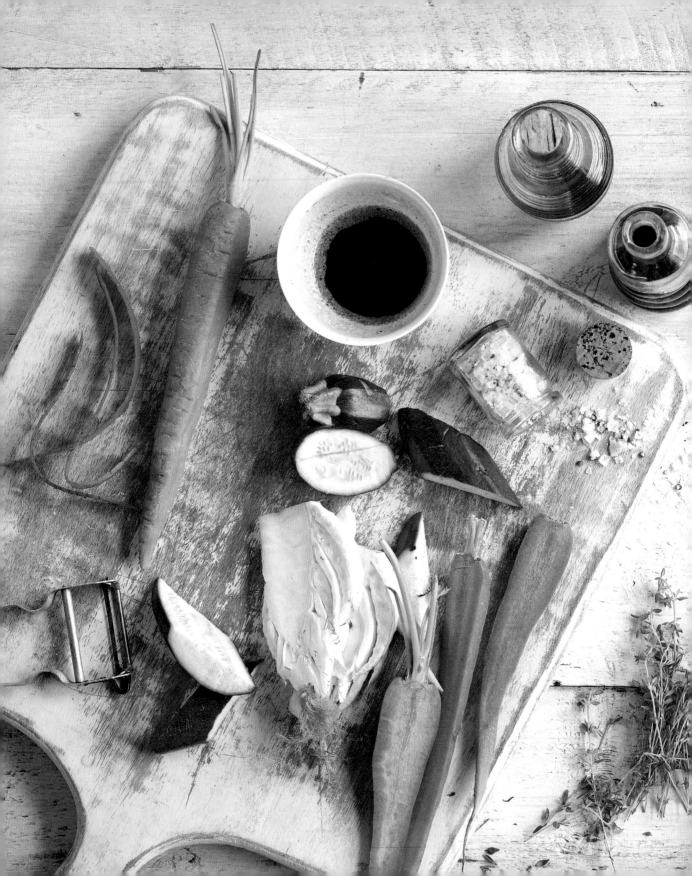

LIGHT MEALS, SNACKS & SIDES

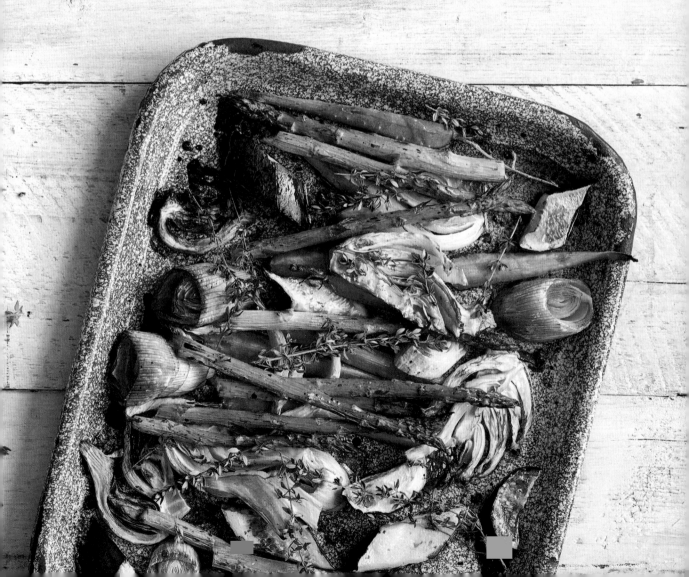

EGG & ZUCCHINI MUFFINS

These make a great protein-packed snack or breakfast. If you want a fluffier, soufflé-type version, beat the egg whites until they form soft peaks, then add the remaining ingredients.

158 CALORIES | 9G FAT | 2.5G SATURATES | 2.5G CARBS | 2G SUGAR | 0.5G SALT | 15G PROTEIN | 1.5G FIBER

- -

SERVES 4

2 cups mesclun, to serve

for the muffins
olive oil spray

6 eggs

3 egg whites

1 large zucchini, coarsely grated

½ red onion, finely chopped

a handful of fresh basil leaves, finely chopped

1 teaspoon crushed black pepper

1. Preheat the oven to 350°F and lightly grease a muffin tin with cooking spray.

2. In a large bowl, beat the eggs well, then add the remaining muffin ingredients, and stir to combine.

3. Pour or spoon the mixture into four muffin cups, almost all the way full, then bake until cooked through or lightly golden, 18 to 20 minutes.

4. Serve with a fresh green salad.

EGG & TUNA MUFFINS

190 CALORIES | 9G FAT | 2.5G SATURATES | 2G CARBS | 2G SUGAR | 0.6G SALT | 22G PROTEIN | 1.2G FIBER

- -

SERVES 4

2 cups mesclun, to serve

for the muffins
olive oil spray

8 white mushrooms, finely chopped

6 eggs

3 egg whites

½ red onion, finely chopped

1 × 5-ounce can water-packed tuna, drained

a handful of fresh basil leaves, finely chopped

1 teaspoon crushed black pepper

1. Preheat the oven to 350°F and lightly grease a muffin tin with cooking spray.

2. Place a non-stick frying pan over medium-high heat, spray with a little oil, and sauté the mushrooms for 2 to 3 minutes until golden brown, then set aside to cool.

3. In a large bowl, beat the eggs well, then add the remaining muffin ingredients, and stir to combine.

4. Pour or spoon the mixture into four muffin cups, almost all the way full, then bake until cooked through or lightly golden, 18 to 20 minutes. Serve with a fresh green salad.

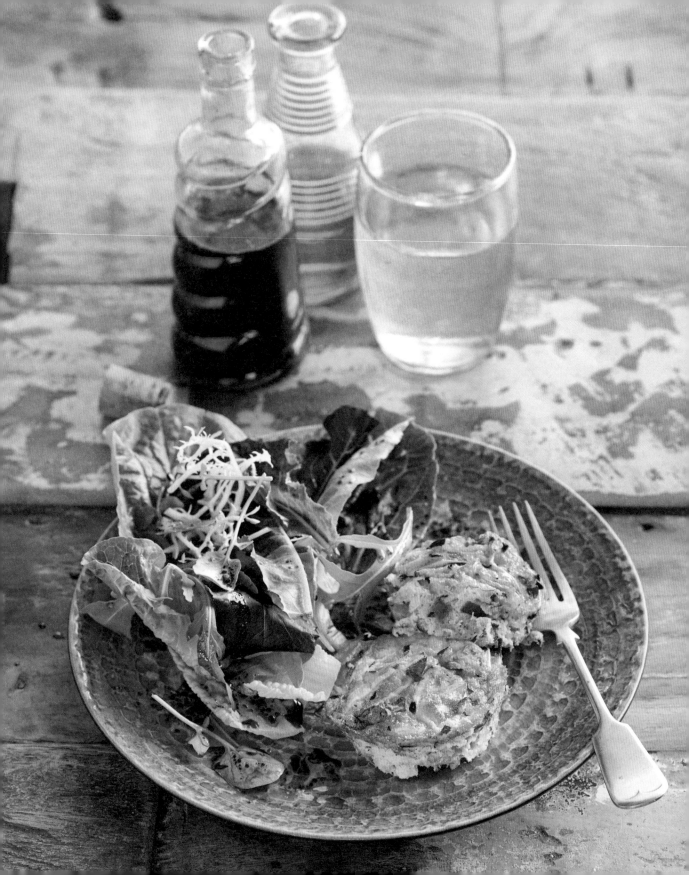

TRUFFLE OIL AVOCADO

This is so simple and yet so tasty, I could eat copious amounts of it all day long (it goes perfectly with either grilled steak or chicken). It also feels like a real indulgence so it's great when you need a treat but don't want to fall off the wagon too hard or too fast.

497 CALORIES | 51G FAT | 9G SATURATES | 3G CARBS | 0.7G SUGAR | 0G SALT | 3G PROTEIN | 7G FIBER

----

1 avocado, peeled and pitted
2 tablespoons white truffle oil
juice of ½ large lemon

1. Place all the ingredients in a food processor (or alternatively use a hand-held electric blender) and process until almost smooth.

2. Serve with crudités or grilled steak or chicken.

AVOCADO MAYO

Commercial mayonnaise is often full of preservatives and offers you very little in terms of nutrition. However, this homemade version using mild-flavored avocado oil is the opposite. It tastes just like traditional mayo but is incredibly healthy and delicious.

918 CALORIES | 99G FAT | 16G SATURATES | 0.5G CARBS | 0.5G SUGAR | 0G SALT | 6G PROTEIN | 0G FIBER

----

2 egg yolks
juice of ½ lemon
½ cup avocado oil
pinch of sea salt and freshly
   ground black pepper

1. Place the egg yolks and lemon juice in a food processor and process briefly to combine, then, with the motor on, begin to pour in the avocado oil very slowly, tablespoon by tablespoon.

2. As the avocado oil gradually mixes in, it will begin to thicken and create a mayo-like consistency. Add more oil as needed to help thicken it even more, then season to taste.

3. Season with salt and pepper and place the mayo in a container and refrigerate.

AVOCADO TOMATILLO SAUCE

This sauce can be served as a dip with crudités or used to spice up any simple fillet of fish, chicken, or beef.

850 CALORIES | 62G FAT | 13G SATURATES | 42G CARBS | 37G SUGAR | 2G SALT | 14G PROTEIN | 33G FIBER

4 fresh tomatillos, peeled

2 avocados, peeled and pitted

3 garlic cloves

juice of 1½ limes

6 to 10 sprigs of fresh cilantro

¼ to ½ teaspoon sea salt

for the crudités

⅔ pound carrots, peeled and cut into sticks

⅔ pound celery, cut into sticks

½ cucumber, cut into sticks

a bunch of breakfast radishes, topped and tailed and quartered

1. Bring a pan of lightly salted water to a boil and cook the tomatillos for about 3 to 4 minutes to soften. Allow to cool.

2. Place all the ingredients for the sauce in a food processor and process until smooth. Serve straight away with crudités.

TIP Tomatillos are also called *tomates verdes* in Mexico (which means green tomatoes) and are a staple in Mexican cooking (their delicious green salsas). They're best when they're about the size of a cherry tomato and have a wonderful citrusy sweet flavor. To prepare, simply stem, remove the papery outer layer, and wash.

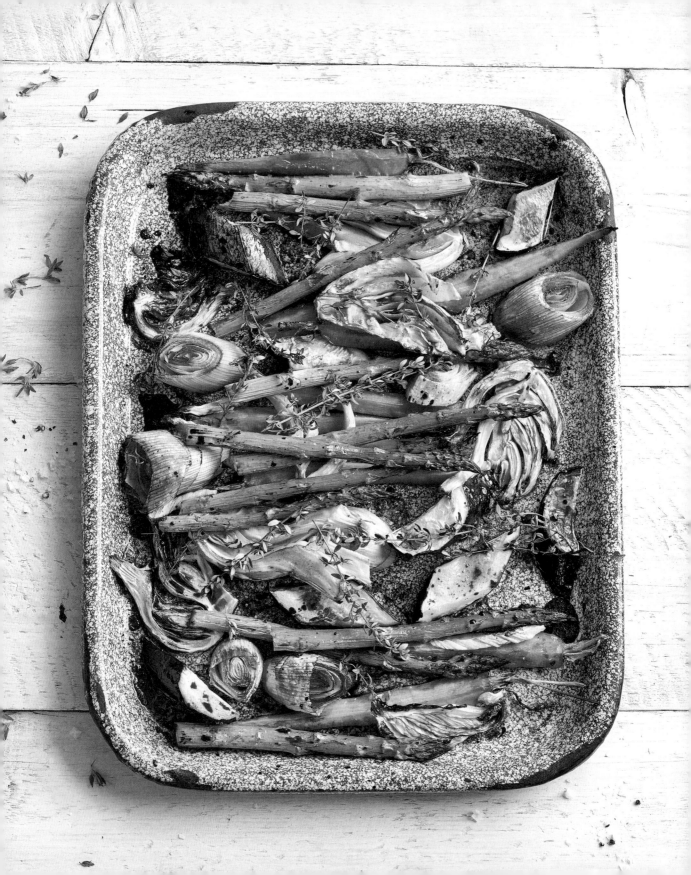

ROASTED VEGETABLES
WITH WHITE TRUFFLE SALT

I think this is one of the easiest, simplest, and best ways to eat vegetables as the roasting brings out their sweet flavor and makes them deliciously tender.

295 CALORIES | 14G FAT | 2G SATURATES | 22G CARBS | 20G SUGAR | 2.7G SALT | 10G PROTEIN | 17G FIBER

SERVES 2 TO 4

¾ pound carrots, topped, tailed and halved lengthways

12 white mushrooms, stems removed

2 leeks, trimmed and sliced

a handful of asparagus, trimmed

1 fennel, cut into wedges

2 zucchini, topped, tailed, halved lengthways, and cut into large chunks

1 tablespoon chopped fresh thyme

2 tablespoons olive oil

1 tablespoon balsamic vinegar

1 teaspoon white truffle salt

1. Preheat the oven to 400°F.

2. In a large bowl, mix the vegetables together with the thyme, olive oil, and vinegar.

3. Tip all the vegetables into a large roasting pan and roast for 10 minutes, then take out of the oven, give the pan a shake, and roast for an additional 10 minutes or until soft, golden, and cooked through.

4. Sprinkle over white truffle salt and serve immediately.

TIP Truffle salt is sea salt infused with the Italian delicacy of dried truffles, which lends it a deliciously rich, earthy flavor. It makes a great alternative seasoning (try it with eggs) and is a great thing to have on hand in your Paleo pantry.

SALMON FISHCAKES
WITH ASIAN DRESSING

This is one of the recipes that I come back to time and time again. I included it in my very first cookbook, back in 2002, but every time I make the recipe, I refine it a little and this version contains even more flavor.

545 CALORIES | 43G FAT | 7.5G SATURATES | 3G CARBS | 2.5G SUGAR | 0.3G SALT | 35G PROTEIN | 2.5G FIBER

SERVES 4

1 tablespoon olive oil,
  for frying
2 cups mesclun, to serve

for the Asian dressing
1-inch piece fresh ginger, grated
¼ cup sesame oil
1 tablespoon sesame seeds
juice of ½ lemon
1 garlic clove, crushed

for the fishcakes
4 × skinless salmon fillets,
  roughly chopped
1 teaspoon sesame oil
1 tablespoon sesame seeds
1 egg
1 egg white
1-inch piece fresh ginger, grated
1 Thai bird's-eye chile, finely
  sliced
4 scallions, finely sliced
½ red onion, finely sliced
a handful of fresh cilantro,
  finely chopped

1. First make the Asian dressing: Simply place all the ingredients in a bowl and whisk well to combine.

2. Now make the fishcakes: Place the salmon, sesame oil, sesame seeds, egg, ginger, chile, scallions, red onion, and cilantro in a food processor and process together, making sure you retain a little texture.

3. On a clean surface, divide the fishcake mixture and carefully shape into little patties about 1-inch thick. Transfer to a plate, cover, and chill for 30 minutes (or up to a day).

4. Heat the olive oil in a large, non-stick sauté pan over high heat and cook about 4 to 5 fish cakes at a time (don't overcrowd the pan or they won't brown up as they should). Cook for a minute, then lower the heat a little, turn and cook for another 60 to 90 seconds (they are small so will cook quickly).

5. Repeat until all the fishcakes are cooked and serve warm, drizzled with a little Asian dressing, and a mesclun salad.

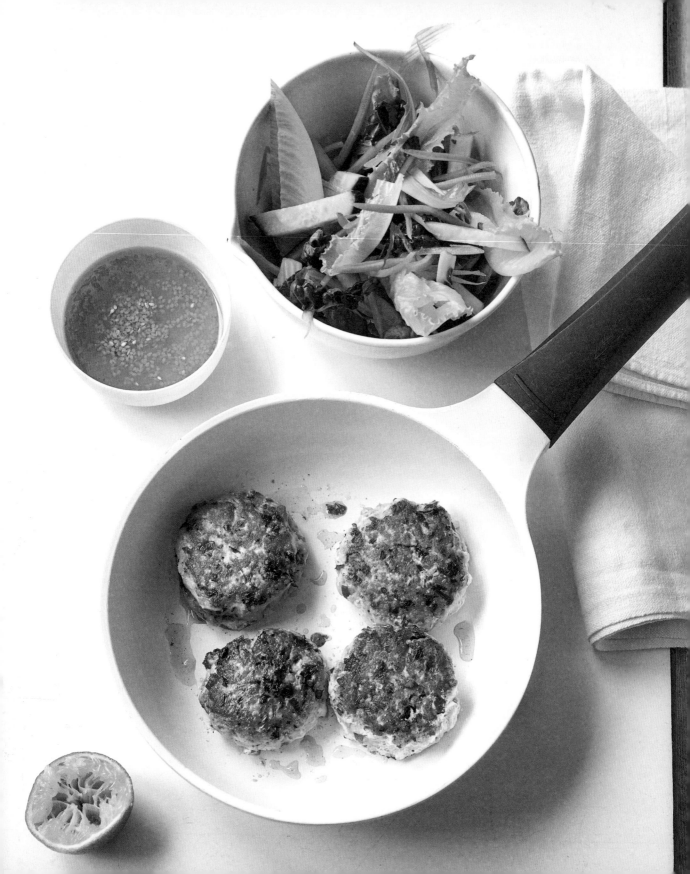

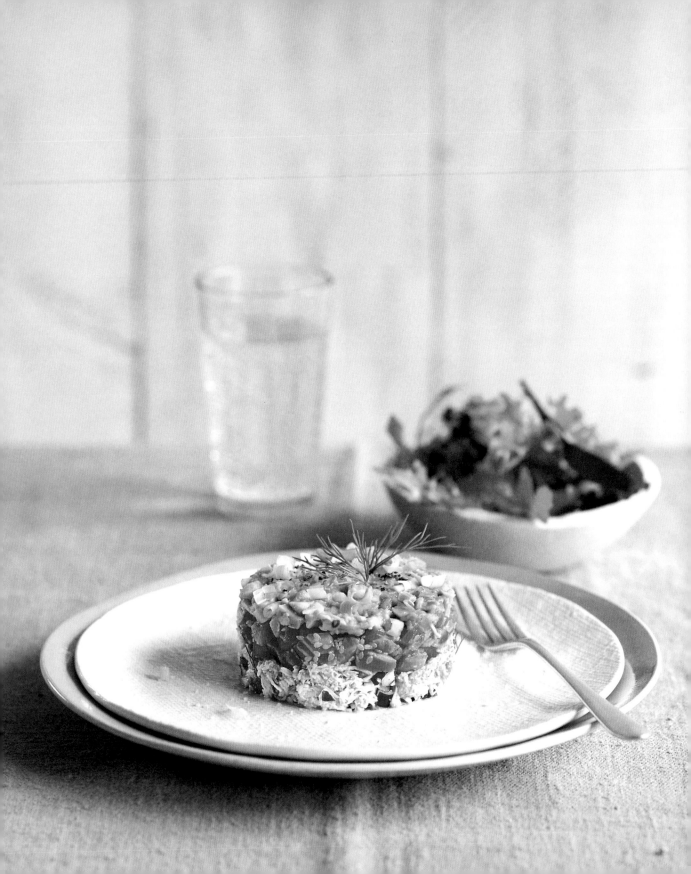

CRAB & SALMON TOWER

This is a great dinner party dish as it's so simple but never fails to impress and no one will ever guess you are on a diet.

452 CALORIES | 30G FAT | 5.5G SATURATES | 3G CARBS | 2G SUGAR | 1.4G SALT | 41G PROTEIN | 3.5G FIBER

SERVES 4

2 × 6-ounce cans crab meat, drained

½ red onion, finely chopped

1 tablespoon olive oil

a handful of fresh dill, roughly chopped

juice of 1 lemon

sea salt and freshly ground black pepper

1 tablespoon sesame seeds

1 pound fresh salmon, cubed (or smoked salmon, finely chopped)

1 avocado, peeled and pitted

a squeeze of lemon

2 scallions, finely chopped

5 ounces (about 4 cups) mesclun

a drizzle of olive oil

1. Place the crab meat in a bowl with the onion, olive oil, dill, and lemon juice. Mix well, season to taste, and set aside.

2. In another bowl, sprinkle the sesame seeds on the salmon and mix until thoroughly coated.

3. In another bowl, mash the avocado with a squeeze of lemon. Season to taste, add the scallions, and mash into the avocado.

4. Place a pastry ring in the center of each plate and spoon in a quarter of the crab mixture, pushing it down well into the mold. Add a layer of avocado and finish with the salmon, pressing everything down so the tower will hold its shape when you remove the pastry ring. Repeat this for each serving.

5. Serve with a fresh green salad, a drizzle of olive oil, and a pinch of salt.

TIP If you want to splurge, substitute fresh crab meat for canned.

SUSHI

Over the following pages, I've included lots and lots of sushi recipes as they are filling and flavorful and full of everything we love about Japanese cuisine, but leaving out the rice makes them almost carb-free, too—perfect for a snack or a lunch on the run.

AVOCADO & SPICY TUNA

314 CALORIES | 18G FAT | 3.5G SATURATES | 3.5G CARBS | 3G SUGAR | 0.2G SALT | 31.5G PROTEIN | 4G FIBER

SERVES 2

½ avocado, chopped into small cubes

½ pound fresh tuna, chopped into small cubes

¼ red onion, finely chopped

1 tablespoon sesame seeds

1 tablespoon sesame oil

¼ red chile, finely chopped (seeded too, if you like)

a handful of fresh cilantro, finely chopped

2 nori (seaweed) sheets

1 scallion, trimmed and sliced lengthways

¼ cucumber, peeled and sliced lengthways into quarters

1. Place the avocado, tuna, red onion, sesame seeds, sesame oil, chile, and cilantro in a bowl and mix together.

2. Lay a nori sheet, shiny side down, on the mat and spread half of the tuna mix across the sheet in a thin layer, but leaving the furthest edge clear.

3. Lay the scallion and cucumber down the middle of each sheet, then use the mat to roll the nori up, applying gentle pressure to keep the roll tight.

4. When you get to the far edge of the nori, dab it with a little water to seal it up. Trim the ends with a sharp knife, then slice the long roll into half, and then half again. Repeat with the second nori sheet, then serve.

TIP A bamboo mat or makisu can be very useful as it helps maintain even pressure from all sides when rolling it up.

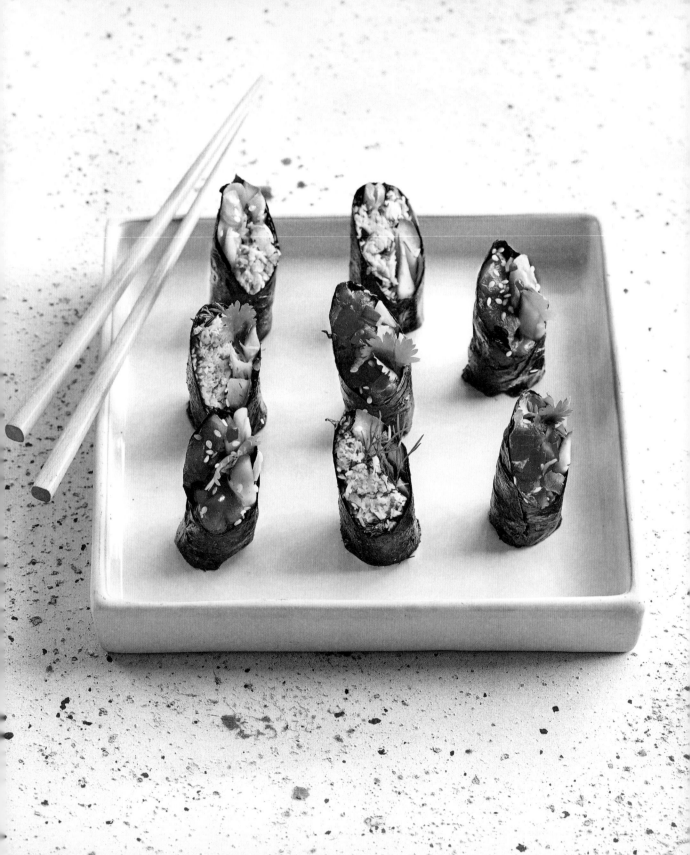

TURKEY & ASPARAGUS

Turkey is so full of protein that one serving (3 ounces) provides 65 percent of your recommended daily intake. It's also packed full of essential amino acids.

309 CALORIES | 5G FAT | 1.5G SATURATES | 4G CARBS | 3G SUGAR | 0.4G SALT | 61G PROTEIN | 3G FIBER

SERVES 2

1 egg

1 pound ground turkey, white meat only (see page 26)

½ red onion, finely chopped

1 garlic clove, crushed

1 teaspoon red pepper flakes

¾-inch piece fresh ginger, grated

a handful of cilantro, finely chopped

4 nori (seaweed) sheets

4 medium asparagus, trimmed

1 jalapeño pepper, trimmed and sliced into rounds

1. Place the egg, ground turkey, onion, garlic, chile, ginger, and cilantro in a bowl and mix together.

2. Lay a nori sheet, shiny side down, on the mat and lay a quarter of the turkey mixture across the sheet in a thin layer, pressing down with a spoon or fork, but leaving the furthest edge clear.

3. Lay the asparagus down the middle of each sheet, then use the mat to roll the nori up, applying gentle pressure to keep the roll tight. When you get to the far edge of the nori, dab it with a little water to seal it up. Repeat with the remaining nori sheets.

4. Place the rolls in a bamboo steamer set over a saucepan of boiling water, turn the heat down to low, and steam for about 22 minutes.

5. Transfer the sushi to a chopping board and, using a sharp knife, trim the ends and then slice the long roll into half, and then half again. Serve each sushi with a slice of jalapeño pepper on top.

CRAB, DILL & ONION

138 CALORIES | 5G FAT | 1G SATURATES | 3.5G CARBS | 3G SUGAR | 1.2G SALT | 18G PROTEIN | 2.5G FIBER

SERVES 2

1 × 6-ounce can white crab meat, drained

¼ red onion, finely chopped

1 tablespoon sesame seeds

1 tablespoon lemon juice

2 tablespoons chopped fresh dill

2 nori (seaweed) sheets

2 scallions, trimmed and
   sliced lengthways

¼ cucumber, peeled and sliced
   lengthways into quarters

1. Place the crab, red onion, sesame seeds, lemon juice, and dill in a bowl and mix together.

2. Lay a nori sheet, shiny side down, on the mat and spread half of the crab mixture across the sheet in a thin layer, but leaving the furthest edge clear.

3. Lay the scallion and cucumber down the middle of each sheet, then use the mat to roll the sushi up, applying gentle pressure to keep the roll tight.

4. When you get to the far edge of the nori, dab it with a little water to seal it up. Trim the ends with a sharp knife, then slice the long roll into half, and then half again. Repeat with the second nori sheet, then serve.

TUNA SALAD WITH WASABI

119 CALORIES | 0.8G FAT | 0G SATURATES | 3G CARBS | 2.5G SUGAR | 0.2G SALT | 24G PROTEIN | 2G FIBER

SERVES 2

1 × 6-ounce can tuna in water, drained

1 teaspoon wasabi paste

¼ red onion, finely chopped

4 to 6 fresh basil leaves, finely sliced

2 nori (seaweed) sheets

1 tablespoon lemon juice

1 scallion

¼ cucumber, peeled and sliced
   lengthways into quarters

1. Place the tuna, red onion, lemon juice, wasabi, and basil in a bowl and mix together.

2. Lay a nori sheet, shiny side down, on the mat and spread half of the tuna mixture across the sheet in a thin layer, but leaving the furthest edge clear.

3. Lay the scallion and cucumber down the middle of each sheet, then use the mat to roll the sushi up, applying gentle pressure to keep the roll tight.

4. When you get to the far edge of the nori, dab it with a little water to seal it up. Trim the ends with a sharp knife, then slice the long roll into half, and then half again. Repeat with the second nori sheet, then serve.

SALMON & SESAME

346 CALORIES | 26G FAT | 4.5G SATURATES | 1.5G CARBS | 1.5G SUGAR | 0.5G SALT | 25G PROTEIN | 4.5G FIBER

SERVES 2

7 ounces salmon fillet

2 nori (seaweed) sheets

1 tablespoon sesame seeds

1 teaspoon sesame oil

7 ounces (about 5 cups) fresh
spinach

1. Place the salmon fillet on a chopping board and, using a very sharp knife, slice lengthways into quarters.

2. Lay a nori sheet, shiny side down, on the mat and place two salmon slices lengthways, edge to edge. Sprinkle over half the sesame seeds and drizzle over half the sesame oil.

3. Wilt the spinach in a bamboo steamer set over a pan of gently simmering water, then squeeze out the excess juices with a sheet of paper towels.

4. Line the spinach next to the salmon along the nori sheet, then then use the mat to roll the sushi up, applying gentle pressure to keep the roll tight.

5. When you get to the far edge, dab it with a little water to seal it up. Trim the ends with a sharp knife, then slice the long roll into half, and then half again. Repeat with the second nori sheet, then serve.

TIP Always ask the fishmonger if the salmon is fresh so you can have it raw. If you are worried about using raw salmon you can squeeze fresh lemon juice over the fish and let it cure for 3 to 4 minutes as this kills most bacteria.

SALMON SASHIMI

270 CALORIES | 17G FAT | 3G SATURATES | 4G CARBS | 3G SUGAR | 1.2G SALT | 24G PROTEIN | 1.7G FIBER

SERVES 2

8 ounces salmon fillet, chopped into cubes

½ yellow onion finely chopped

1 tablespoon coconut aminos

¼ red chile, finely chopped (seeded if you like)

juice of 1 lemon

2 nori (seaweed) sheets

¼ cucumber, peeled and sliced lengthways into quarters

1. Place the salmon, onion, coconut aminos, chile, and lemon juice in a bowl and mix together.

2. Lay a nori sheet, shiny side down, on the mat and spread half of the salmon mixture across the sheet in a thin layer, but leaving the furthest edge clear.

3. Lay the cucumber down the middle of each sheet, then use the mat to roll the sushi up, applying gentle pressure to keep the roll tight.

4. When you get to the far edge of the nori, dab it with a little water to seal it up. Trim the ends with a sharp knife, then slice the long roll into half, and then half again. Repeat with the second nori sheet, then serve.

TUNA SASHIMI

368 CALORIES | 11.5G FAT | 2G SATURATES | 0.8G CARBS | 0.6G SUGAR | 0.6G SALT | 61G PROTEIN | 7G FIBER

SERVES 2

1 pound tuna, finely cubed

¼ red onion, finely chopped

a handful of fresh cilantro, roughly chopped

1 tablespoon sesame oil

1 tablespoon sesame seeds

¼ red chile, finely chopped

¾-inch piece fresh ginger, grated

¼ cucumber, finely chopped

wasabi paste (see page 68)

4 nori (seaweed) sheets

1. Place all the ingredients except the wasabi and seaweed in a bowl and mix well.

2. Lay a nori sheet, shiny side down, on the mat and draw a thin line of wasabi paste across the length of the sheet. Spread a quarter of the tuna mixture across the sheet in a thin layer, leaving the furthest edge clear, and use the mat to roll the sushi up, applying gentle pressure to keep the roll tight.

3. When you get to the far edge of the nori, dab it with a little water to seal it up. Trim the ends with a sharp knife, then slice the long roll into half, and then half again. Repeat with the remaining nori sheets, then serve.

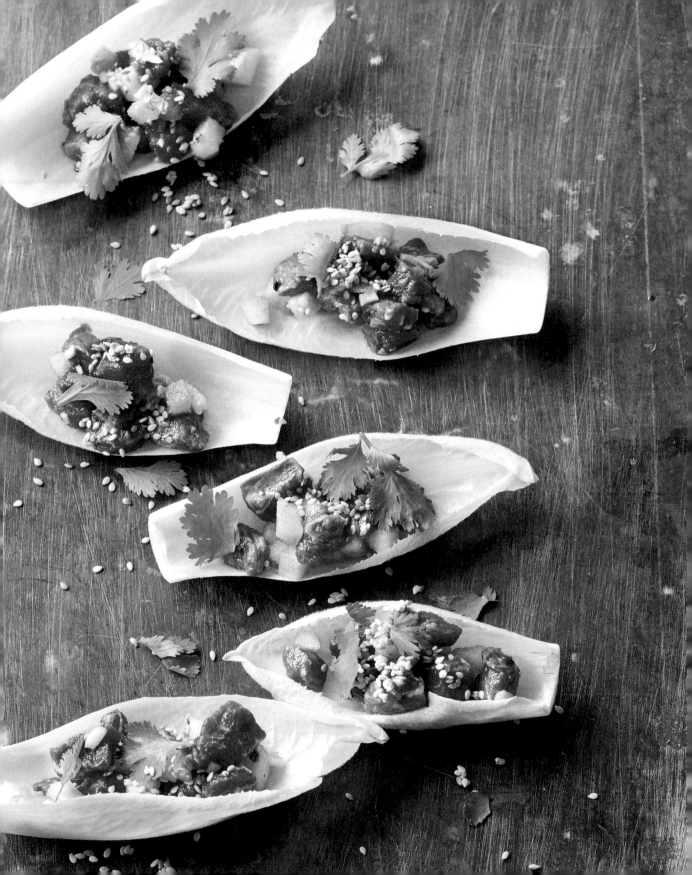

KOREAN BEEF TARTARE

I first tasted this staple Korean dish when I was in Seoul and it blew me away. The traditional version does use a lot of soy sauce, which is not strictly a Paleo ingredient. However, coconut aminos provide a very good soy sauce substitute (see page 10) so try it and see what you think.

433 CALORIES | 17.5G FAT | 5G SATURATES | 14G CARBS | 11.5G SUGAR | 1G SALT | 54G PROTEIN | 1.5G FIBER

SERVES 4

1 Asian (Nashi) pear, peeled, cored, and sliced into thin strips

juice of ½ lemon

2 pounds very lean beef (beef tenderloin is best)

3 garlic cloves, finely chopped

2 tablespoons sesame oil

1 tablespoon sesame seeds

3 tablespoons coconut aminos (see page 10)

2 tablespoons raw honey or maple syrup

2 heads Belgian endive, leaves separated

a handful of flat-leaf parsley, finely chopped

1. Place the Asian pear in a small bowl and squeeze over the lemon juice to prevent it from discoloring, then place in the fridge.

2. Cut the beef tenderloin into very small pieces and place in a large bowl. If you find any fat, discard it. Add the garlic, sesame oil, sesame seeds, and coconut aminos to the beef and mix well. Add the honey and mix again until thoroughly combined. Cover and refrigerate for at least 20 minutes, but no more than an hour.

3. When ready to serve, add the pear to the beef and mix again. Serve with a few Belgian endive leaves and a sprinkling of parsley to garnish.

TIP I recommend that you use beef tenderloin for this recipe and do make sure that the meat is very very fresh as you are serving it raw.

OLIVE & TUNA TAPENADE

347 CALORIES | 20G FAT | 3G SATURATES | 15G CARBS | 14G SUGAR | 3.3G SALT | 22G PROTEIN | 11G FIBER

SERVES 2

for the dip
1 × 6-ounce can pitted black olives
1 × 5-ounce can water-packed tuna, drained
1 tablespoon capers
1 tablespoon olive oil
1 garlic clove, peeled
juice of ½ lemon
½ yellow onion
a small handful of fresh basil (optional)
1 tablespoon Dijon mustard

for the crudités
⅔ pound carrots, peeled and cut into sticks
⅔ pound celery, cut into sticks
½ cucumber, cut into sticks
a bunch of radishes, topped and tailed and quartered

1. Simply place all the dip ingredients in a food processor (or alternatively use a hand-held electric blender) and whiz together for a few minutes, ensuring the ingredients are chopped but still nice and chunky (this is a tapenade, not a paste).

2. Serve as a dip with a selection of fresh, crunchy crudités.

SALMON TAPENADE

285 CALORIES | 12G FAT | 2G SATURATES | 15G CARBS | 13G SUGAR | 1.6G SALT | 25G PROTEIN | 8G FIBER

SERVES 2

for the dip
1 × 6-ounce can salmon, drained
juice of 1 lemon
1 teaspoon capers
a small handful of fresh basil leaves
1 tablespoon sun-dried tomatoes in olive oil
4 to 6 cherry tomatoes
½ small red chile or 1 teaspoon red pepper flakes
¼ red onion, finely chopped
a few chives, chopped (for garnish)

for the crudités
⅔ pound carrots, peeled and cut into sticks
⅔ pound celery, cut into sticks
½ cucumber, cut into sticks
a bunch of radishes, topped and tailed and quartered

1. Place all the dip ingredients except the red onion and chives in a food processor and process until it is a nice chunky blend, then transfer to a bowl.

2. Add the red onion and stir through and serve with crudités of your choice with a sprinkle of chopped chives.

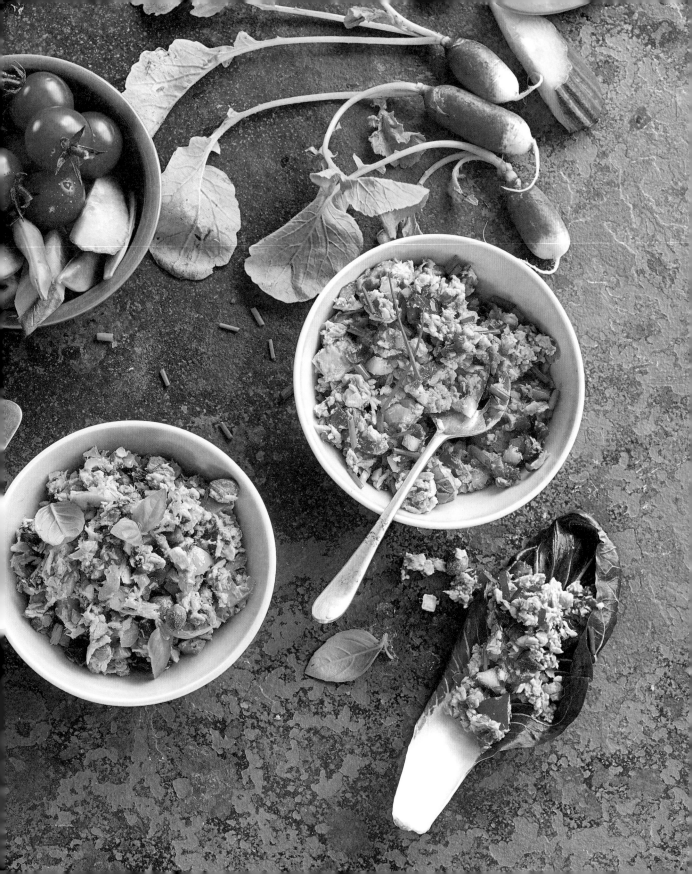

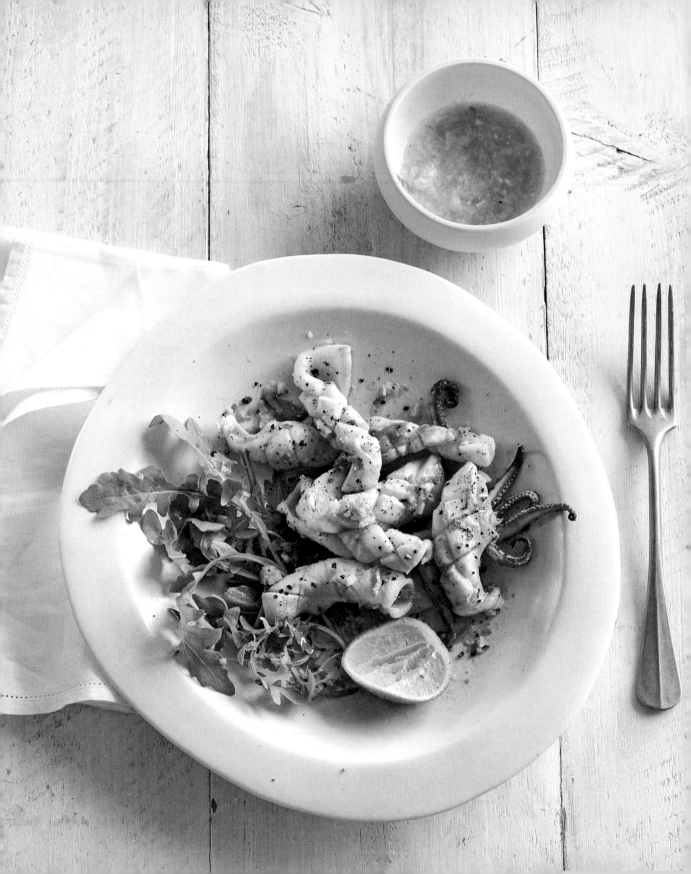

PAN-FRIED CALAMARI
WITH GINGER & LIME

When we think of calamari we often think of deep-fried guilty pleasure. However, with this recipe you can skip the guilt and just focus on the pleasure. Squid is also very inexpensive, plus it's full of protein and essential vitamins and minerals (especially calcium).

212 CALORIES | 7G FAT | 1.5G SATURATES | 1G CARBS | 1G SUGAR | 0.6G SALT | 36G PROTEIN | 1.5G

SERVES 4

1 tablespoon olive oil

2 pounds squid, cleaned and thinly sliced

sea salt and freshly ground black pepper

zest of ½ lime

juice of 1 lime

2 garlic cloves, crushed

1-inch piece fresh ginger, grated

14 ounces (about 5 cups) arugula

1 lemon, quartered

1. Place the olive oil in a large non-stick frying pan and place over very high heat. When hot, add the squid, season and stir-fry for 3 to 4 minutes, then transfer to a bowl, being sure to include all the crispy pan scrapings and set aside.

2. In a bowl, mix together the lime zest, lime juice, garlic, and ginger.

3. Arrange a pile of arugula on a plate, place the calamari on top with the lemon wedges, then pour over the citrusy sauce.

TIP You can add a little extra virgin olive oil when you plate the dish, and a twist of freshly ground black pepper.

SALMON & SCALLOP CEVICHE

This is such a healthy, fresh-tasting dish and it looks so beautiful arranged on one big serving plate—a dinner party starter that's perfect for sharing. Feel free to add a little wasabi, if you like.

267 CALORIES | 16.5G FAT | 3G SATURATES | 2G CARBS | 1.5G SUGAR | 0.3G SALT | 27G PROTEIN | 0.7G

SERVES 4

12 ounces skinless salmon fillet

8 large scallops

juice of ½ lime

1 tablespoon olive oil

1 small red chile, seeded and finely chopped

6 chives, finely chopped

4 shallots, finely chopped

sea salt and freshly ground black pepper

wasabi paste, optional

1. Using a very sharp knife, cut the salmon and scallops into very thin slices.

2. Arrange the fish and seafood on a plate and squeeze over the lime juice, then drizzle with olive oil.

3. Place the chile, chives, and shallots in a bowl and mix together well, then sprinkle the ceviche on the plate. Season with salt and pepper and serve immediately with a little wasabi if desired.

TIP If you are a little concerned about cooking with raw fish at home, don't be put off by this recipe as the acidity of the lime juice cures the salmon and scallops, which eliminates any bacteria. However, it is always best to use the freshest fish and seafood you can find and I recommend asking your fishmonger so you are absolutely sure.

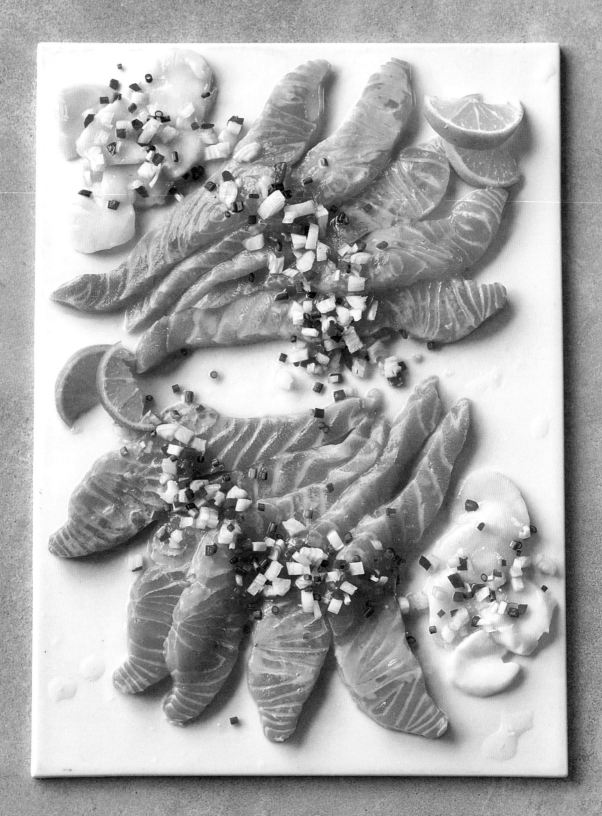

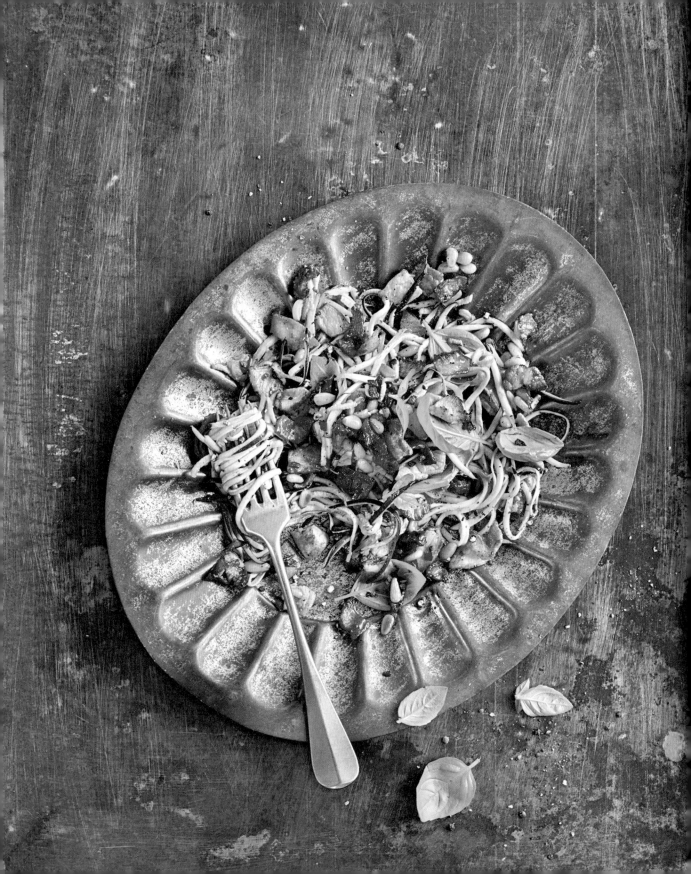

ZUCCHINI SPAGHETTI
WITH BACON & BASIL

This recipe gives you the texture and flavor of spaghetti but without the carbs—genius! And if you want to make the best, long zucchini spaghetti ribbons it's a good idea to invest in a julienne peeler or a fancy spiralizing gadget.

208 CALORIES | 17G FAT | 3.5G SATURATES | 3G CARBS | 3G SUGAR | 1.1G SALT | 9.5G PROTEIN | 2G FIBER

- -

SERVES 4 AS A SNACK OR SIDE DISH TO ANY MAIN MEAL

4 zucchini

2 tablespoons olive oil

6 slices Canadian bacon, trimmed of all fat and thinly sliced

1 garlic clove, crushed

¾ cup sun-dried tomatoes in olive oil, drained and sliced into strips

1 small red chile, finely chopped

1 tablespoon pine nuts

a handful of fresh basil, thinly shredded

1. First make your spaghetti by either grating the zucchini at an angle on the largest side of a cheese grater or using a hand-held julienne peeler or spiralizer.

2. Place 1 tablespoon olive oil in a large non-stick frying pan over high heat and stir-fry the zucchini for 3 minutes. Add the bacon to the pan and sauté for a few minutes until cooked. Reduce the heat to medium.

3. Add the garlic, sun-dried tomatoes, chile, pine nuts, and the remaining olive oil to the pan. Toss for a few minutes, then take off the heat.

4. Divide the spaghetti between four bowls, sprinkle with the basil, and serve immediately.

- -

TIP To prevent the zucchini spaghetti from getting mushy, either cook it in a very large pan or do it in two batches.

TUNA TATAKI

Nothing is more Paleo than a beautiful plate of fresh, raw fish. I also love making this with salmon, and sometimes, instead of shredding the seaweed, I enclose the fish in a nori wrap.

421 CALORIES | 16G FAT | 3.5G SATURATES | 2.5G CARBS | 1.5G SUGAR | 0.9G SALT | 65G PROTEIN | 3G FIBER

SERVES 4

2.2 pounds very fresh tuna

½ small red onion, finely chopped

a handful of fresh cilantro leaves, finely chopped

1 tablespoon coconut aminos

1 tablespoon sesame seeds

1-inch piece fresh ginger, grated

1 tablespoon sesame oil

1 red bird's-eye chile, finely chopped

1 sheet of seaweed, shredded

1 large avocado, diced

1. With a very sharp knife, on a very clean chopping board, shave the tuna into long, thin slices, discarding any sinew. Transfer to a bowl.

2. Add all the remaining ingredients to the bowl and mix well. Finally stir through the avocado and divide between four plates.

3. Serve with an extra sprinkle of cilantro.

TIP The B vitamins in tuna help to build and maintain red blood cells and increase energy. They also increase the rate of metabolism, strengthen the immune system, and keep the skin healthy.

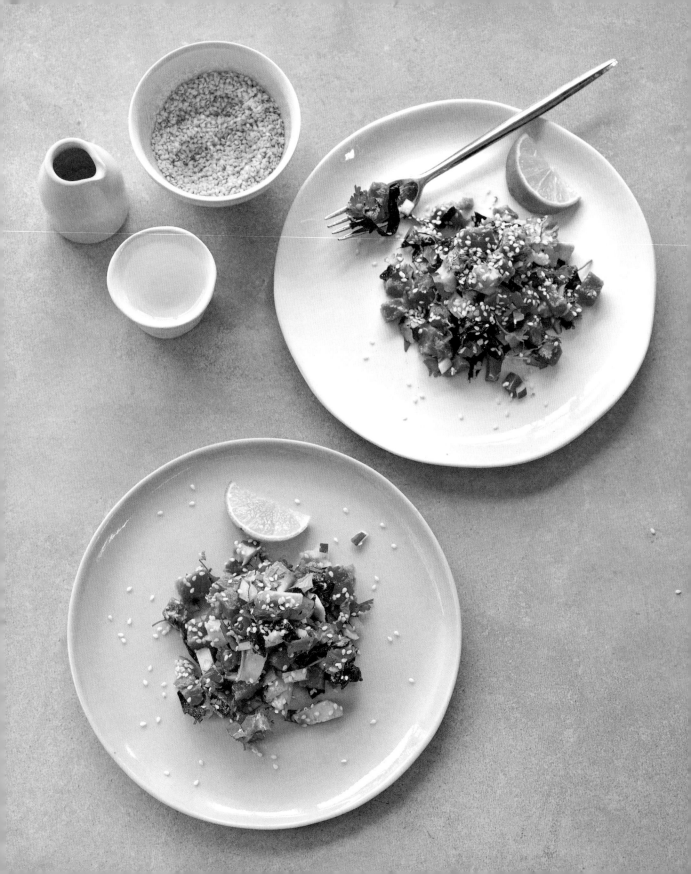

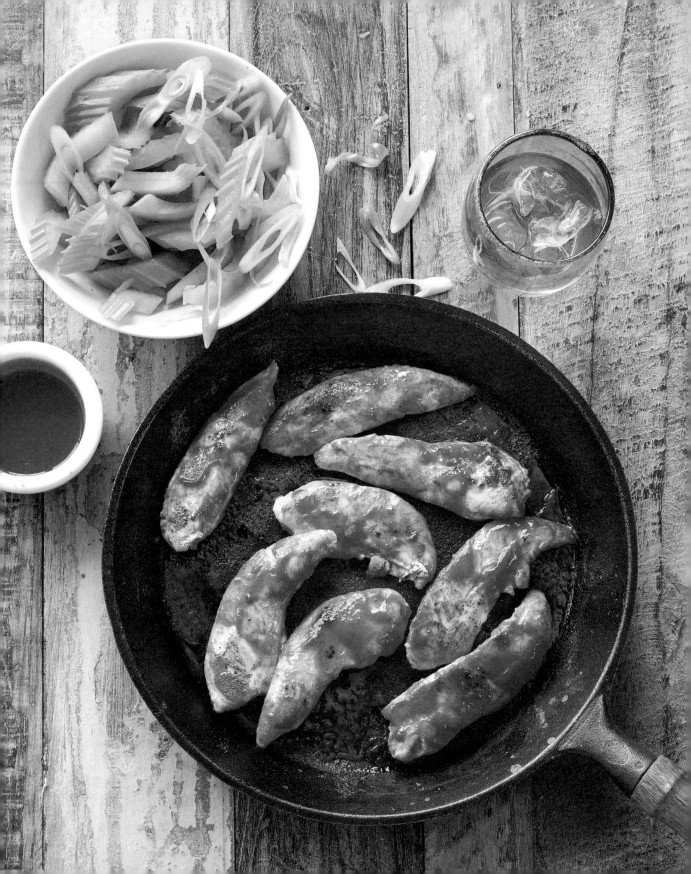

BUFFALO CHICKEN STRIPS

Buffalo wings are often served as starters or bar food and, more often than not, they're deep-fried and served with blue cheese dip—delicious, but perhaps not one of the healthiest foods out there! My version, however, is healthy and sacrifices none of the flavor. You really do have to use Frank's sauce for authenticity but as it contains a few ingredients that aren't strictly Paleo, keep this for a weekend, or alternatively make up your own Hot Wings Sauce using the recipe below.

377 CALORIES | 14G FAT | 8G SATURATES | 2G CARBS | 2G SUGAR | 0.9G SALT | 60G PROTEIN | 1G FIBER

SERVES 4

4 × 8¾-ounce skinless chicken breasts, cut into strips

1 tablespoon olive oil

sea salt and freshly ground black pepper

½ cup buffalo sauce (Frank's Hot Wings Sauce is the one to use, or see the Tip below)

6 large celery sticks, trimmed and finely sliced

4 scallions, finely sliced

1. Rub the chicken strips all over with the olive oil and season lightly.

2. Place a large non-stick frying pan over high heat and cook the chicken for about 3 to 4 minutes on each side. Add the buffalo sauce, then quickly take off the heat (it will bubble fast and the pepper will hit the air), and toss the pan to evenly coat the chicken.

3. Serve the chicken over the celery and sprinkle the scallions on top.

TIP As with so many storebought condiments, Frank's Hot Wings Sauce doesn't quite meet the strict Paleo criteria, so here's a recipe you can make up at home: Melt 3 tablespoons coconut oil in a saucepan over low heat, then whisk in 3 to 4 tablespoons Tabasco, 1 teaspoon garlic powder, 1 teaspoon paprika, 1 tablespoon lemon juice, 1 tablespoon white wine vinegar, and lightly season with salt and pepper.

MEATLOAF

Now that I've been living in the US for over a decade, I've lost count of the incredibly delicious meatloaves that I've tasted over the years. As it's such a classic and staple dish here and as it's the perfect solution for when you're catering for large numbers, I felt I had to include my own Paleo version.

673 CALORIES | 32G FAT | 10G SATURATES | 3.5G CARBS | 2.5G SUGAR | 0.4G SALT | 34G PROTEIN | 1G FIBER

SERVES 8

2 cups salad leaves, to serve

for the meatloaf

2½ pounds lean ground beef

1 egg and 1 egg white

½ yellow onion, finely chopped

3 garlic cloves, crushed

2 tablespoons homemade Hot Wings Sauce (see page 75)

2 to 3 tablespoons freshly chopped parsley

2 tablespoons ground almonds

2 tablespoons tomato paste

2 tablespoons homemade tomato ketchup (see page 26)

¾ cup roughly chopped sun-dried tomatoes

1. Preheat the oven to 350°F.

2. Place all the meatloaf ingredients in a large bowl and, using your hands, mix everything together until thoroughly combined.

3. Take a loaf pan and spray with a little olive oil.

4. Tip the meatloaf mixture into the pan so that it fills every corner, smooth the top and cover with foil. Bake in the oven for 30 minutes, then remove the foil and bake for an additional 20 minutes until beautifully browned on top.

5. Serve hot with something bright and green like a salad.

TIP A pan of hot water in the oven, under the tin, will stop the top of the loaf from cracking.

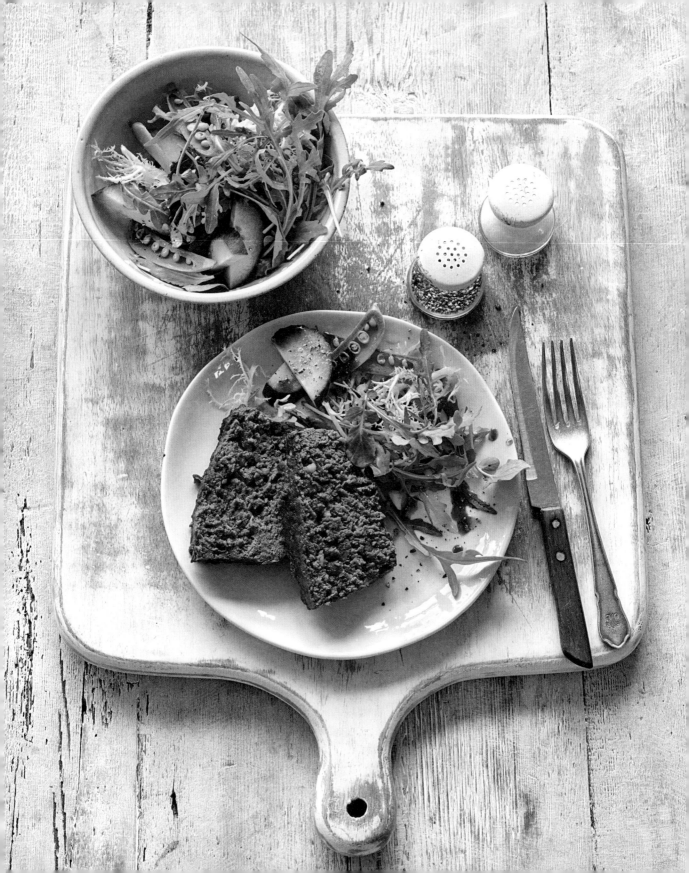

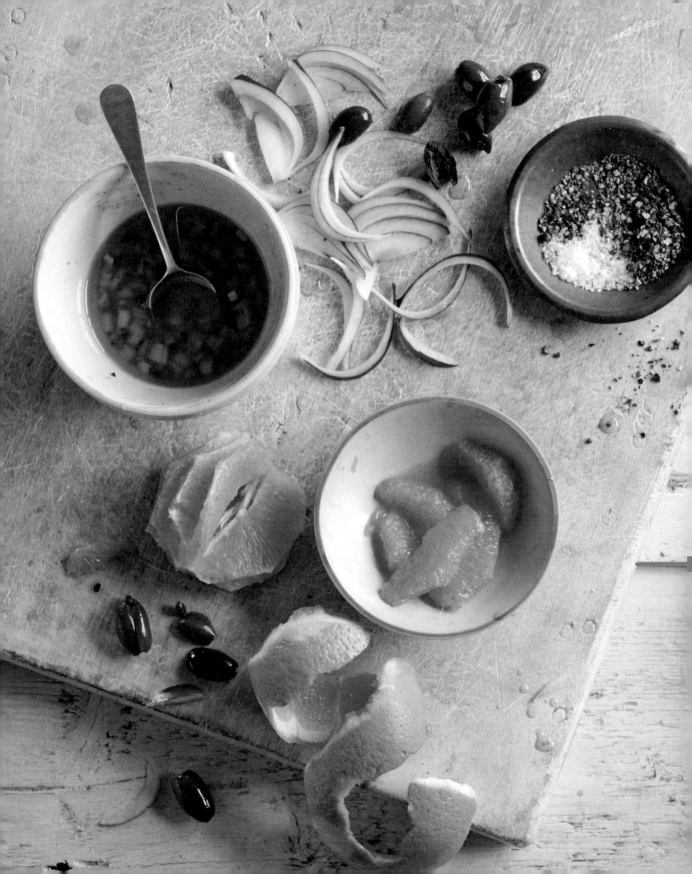

SOUPS & SALADS

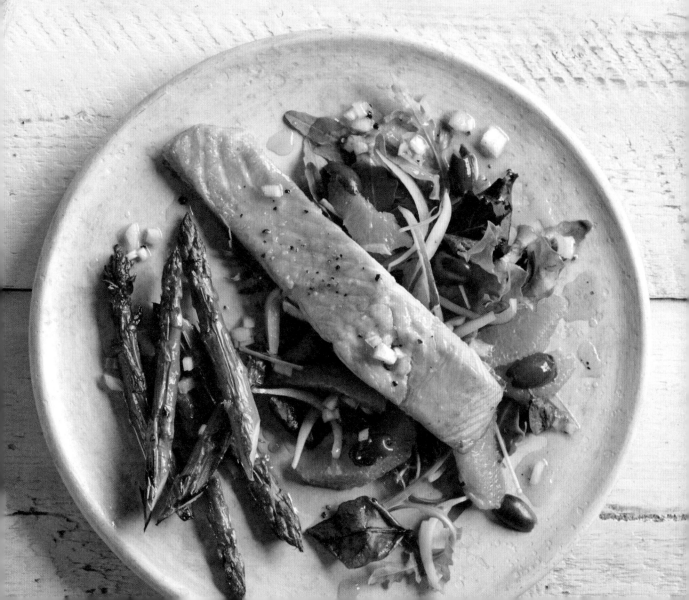

TOMATO SOUP

This is a great example of how you only need a few ingredients to make a fantastic soup and how there's no need for traditional starchy thickeners like potato.

216 CALORIES | 11G FAT | 1.5G SATURATES | 21G CARBS | 20G SUGAR | 1G SALT | 4.5G PROTEIN | 7G FIBER

SERVES 4

1 tablespoon olive oil

2.2 pounds fresh tomatoes

1 cup puréed tomatoes

1 cup vegetable stock

1 cup sun-dried tomatoes in olive oil

1 teaspoon cracked black pepper, plus more to finish

½ teaspoon chile powder

2 garlic cloves, crushed

a handful of fresh basil leaves, shredded

1. Heat the olive oil in a large saucepan over medium heat and sauté the tomatoes for 2 to 3 minutes.

2. Add the puréed tomatoes, stock, and sun-dried tomatoes and stir to combine, then add the pepper, chile and garlic and stir some more.

3. Bring to a boil, cover and simmer for 15 minutes, then add half the basil, stir, and remove from the heat.

4. Using a hand-held immersion blender, purée the soup until smooth, then pour the soup into a saucepan, season with more black pepper, and heat until barely simmering.

5. Remove from the heat, divide between four serving bowls, and garnish with the remaining fresh basil.

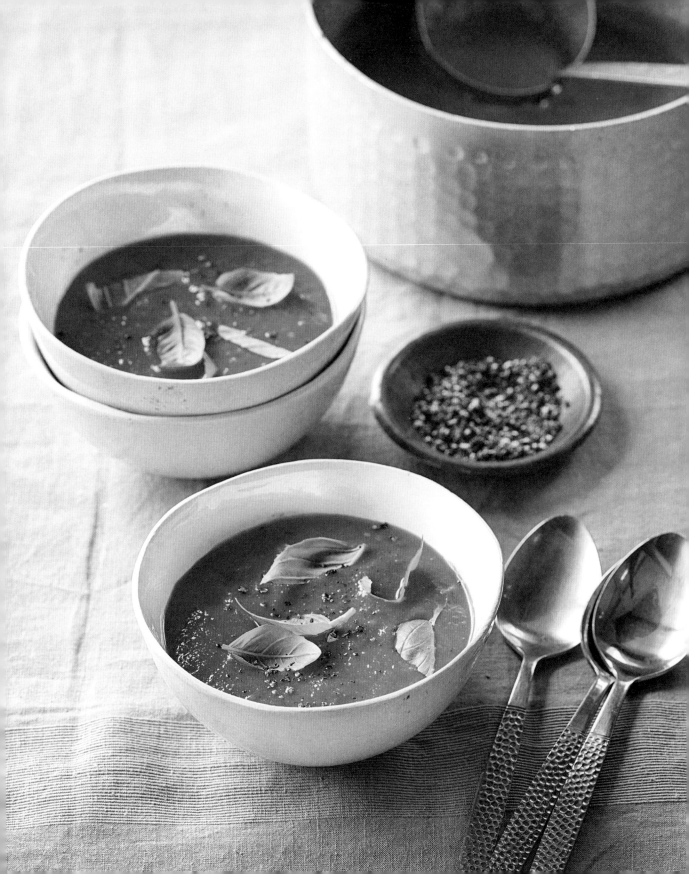

BROCCOLI SOUP

Many soup recipes use potato since the starch works as a great thickening agent. However, there are ingredients, such as watercress or broccoli, which do the same thing without the starch and so are perfect for Paleo.

116 CALORIES | 4G FAT | 0.7G SATURATES | 7.5G CARBS | 5.5G SUGAR | 1.5G SALT | 8G PROTEIN | 8G FIBER

- -

SERVES 4

1 tablespoon olive oil

1 medium yellow onion, roughly chopped

1 medium leek, trimmed and roughly chopped

3 garlic cloves, crushed

1.3 pounds fresh broccoli florets

4 cups vegetable stock

freshly ground black pepper

a handful of basil leaves, torn

1. Heat the oil in a large saucepan over medium heat and sweat the onion for 2 to 3 minutes.

2. Add the leeks and garlic and cook for an additional minute, then add the broccoli and stock, and stir to combine. Turn up the heat to bring to a boil, then reduce to a simmer, and cook for 30 minutes. Set aside to cool.

3. Using a hand-held immersion blender, purée the mixture until smooth.

4. Pour the soup back into the saucepan, season with black pepper, then heat until barely simmering.

5. Remove from the heat, divide between four serving bowls, and garnish with a sprinkling of basil leaves.

- -

TIP If you like a little more texture in your soup, only roughly blend the vegetables so it's not completely smooth.

CAULIFLOWER SOUP

Cauliflower is a great low-carb alternative to using potato as a thickening agent.
Add more stock to this one if you prefer a thinner, more purée-like consistency.

126 CALORIES | 6G FAT | 1G SATURATES | 10G CARBS | 7G SUGAR | 0.1G SALT | 5G PROTEIN | 4G FIBER

SERVES 4

2 tablespoons olive oil

1 medium yellow onion,
　roughly chopped

2 garlic cloves, crushed

1 cauliflower, broken into
　florets

¼ cup vegetable stock

freshly ground black pepper

a handful of flat-leaf parsley,
　finely chopped

1. Heat the olive oil in a large saucepan over medium heat and sweat the onion for 12 minutes.

2. Add the garlic and cauliflower and stir to cook for 1 minute, then cover with stock, bring to a boil, and simmer for 40 minutes. Remove from the heat.

3. Using a hand-held immersion blender, purée until smooth.

4. Pour the soup back into the saucepan, season with black pepper, then heat until barely simmering.

5. Remove from the heat, divide between your serving bowls, and garnish with a sprinkling of parsley.

TIP I love cauliflower as its mild flavor makes it incredibly versatile. Use it as a thickening agent in soups or even cook it until soft and then mash as a wonderful low-carb alternative to mashed potatoes.

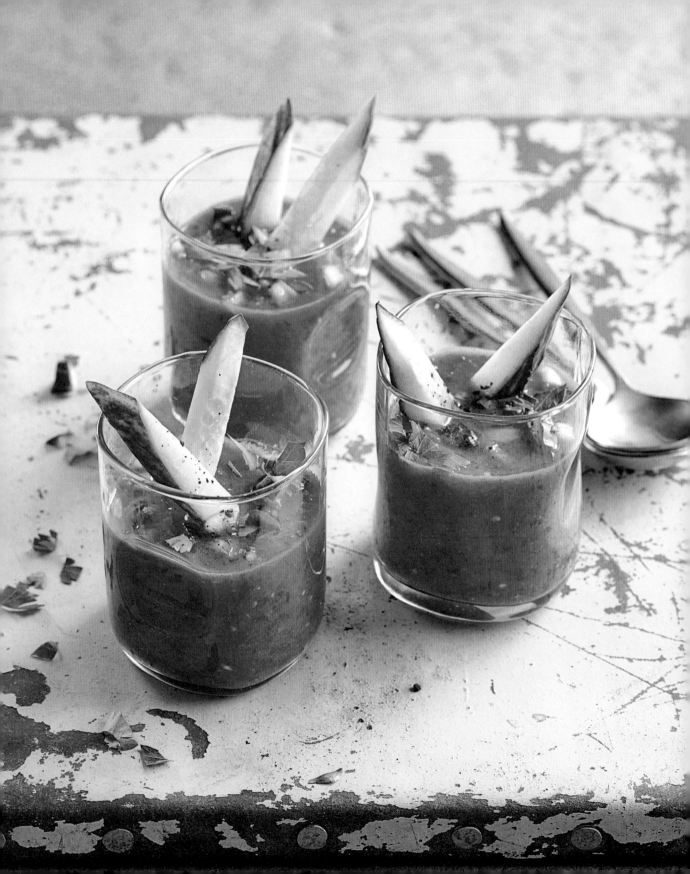

GAZPACHO

This traditional Spanish soup is always served chilled and makes a deliciously refreshing meal in hot weather. Try it in little glasses with shrimp for a summer party canapé.

113 CALORIES | 6G FAT | 0.9G SATURATES | 11G CARBS | 10G SUGAR | TRACE SALT | 2G PROTEIN | 0.4G FIBER

- -

SERVES 4

2.2 pounds tomatoes, roughly chopped

1 small yellow onion, roughly chopped

1 garlic clove, crushed

1 red pepper, seeded and finely chopped

2 tablespoons olive oil

2 tablespoons white wine vinegar

½ cucumber, halved, seeds scooped out, and finely chopped

sea salt and freshly ground black pepper

a handful of flat-leaf parsley, finely chopped

1. Place the tomatoes, onion, garlic, pepper, olive oil, and vinegar in a blender and pulse until smooth. Stir in the cucumber, season to taste, then place in the refrigerator for at least an hour.

2. Serve with a sprinkling of fresh parsley.

- -

TIP This soup also makes a great base for a seafood sauce or a simple fish stew.

VEGETABLE COMFORT SOUP
WITH MEATBALLS

This is my favorite comfort soup for rainy days. It's what I make when I am home all day and feel just plain hungry and however much I eat, it always leaves me feeling satisfied and never like I've overindulged!

293 CALORIES | 7G FAT | 1.7G SATURATES | 10G CARBS | 8G SUGAR | 1G SALT | 46G PROTEIN | 5G FIBER

SERVES 4

for the meatballs
1 pound ground chicken
1 small red chile, finely chopped
½ red onion, finely chopped
1 egg
1 tablespoon tomato paste
4 garlic cloves, crushed
1 tablespoon dried basil

1 tablespoon olive oil
1 medium yellow onion, finely chopped
½ pound carrots, peeled and chopped into small cubes
1 leek, finely chopped
7 cups chicken stock
1 teaspoon freshly ground black pepper
7 ounces (about 5 cups) fresh spinach

1. First make the meatballs: Place the ground chicken, chile, red onion, egg, tomato paste, half the garlic, and half the dried basil in a large bowl and use your hands to mix together well.

2. Divide the mixture into tablespoon-size scoops and roll into balls. Place on a large plate.

3. Heat the oil in a large stockpot and sauté the onion for 2 minutes. Add the carrots, leek, and the remaining basil and garlic, and sauté for an additional minute, then add the stock and pepper and bring to a boil.

4. Add the meatballs to the stockpot, cover, and cook for 15 minutes. Add the spinach, cover again, and cook for an additional 5 minutes.

5. Remove the pan from the heat, divide between four serving bowls, and serve immediately.

TIP If you want a little more flavor, add a tablespoon of homemade pesto.

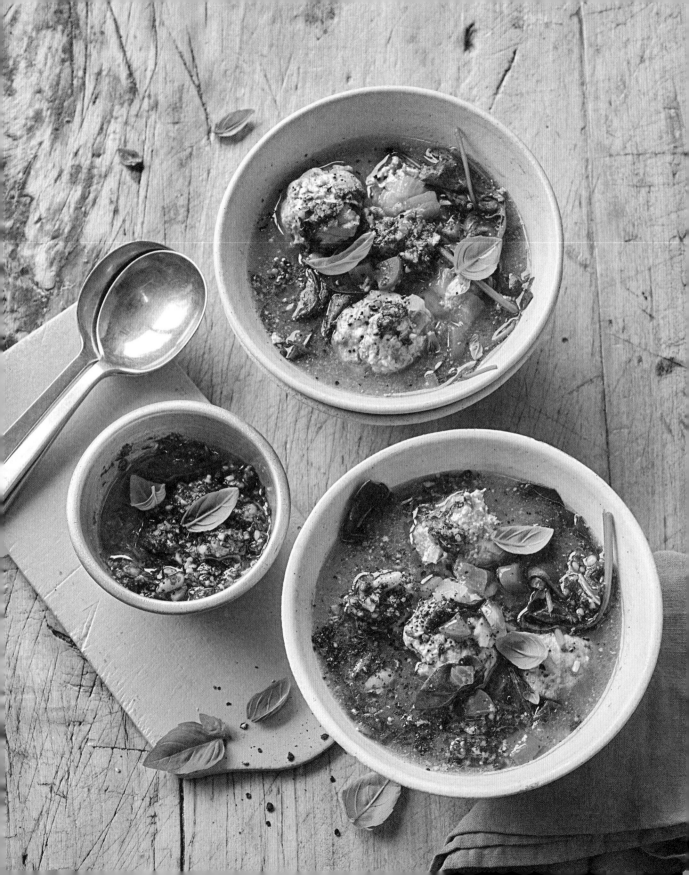

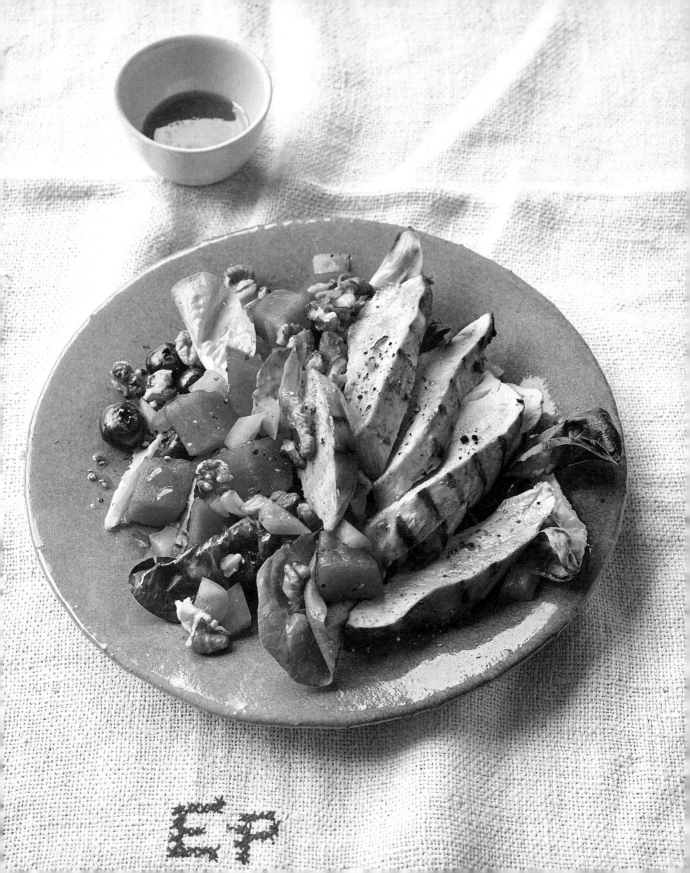

GRILLED CHICKEN SALAD
WITH FRUIT & NUTS

I love including fruit in a salad. It provides such great color and adds a lovely fresh sweetness that works so well with peppery greens and toasted nuts.

247 CALORIES | 8G FAT | 1G SATURATES | 12G CARBS | 12G SUGAR | 0.4G SALT | 30G PROTEIN | 2.5G FIBER

SERVES 4

4 × 4-ounce boneless skinless chicken breast halves

for the marinade
½ cup fresh lime juice
2 tablespoons honey
4 teaspoons olive oil
½ teaspoon salt
½ teaspoon pepper

for the salad
5 ounces (about 5 cups) mixed salad greens
1 cup cubed seedless watermelon
1½ cups fresh blueberries
1 medium yellow pepper, cubed
2 tablespoons chopped walnuts, toasted

1. First make the marinade: In a small bowl, combine the lime juice, honey, oil, salt, and pepper and whisk together.

2. Pour two-thirds of the marinade into a large resealable plastic bag. Place the chicken in the bag, seal it and, ensuring all the meat is covered with the marinade, place in the fridge for at least 1 hour. Set the remaining marinade mixture aside for a dressing.

3. When you are ready to cook the chicken, heat a grill pan over medium heat. When hot, drain and discard the marinade and cook the chicken in the hot pan for 4 to 7 minutes on each side.

4. In a large bowl, combine the salad greens, watermelon, blueberries, and yellow pepper, add the reserved dressing, and toss to coat. Divide among four serving plates.

5. Using a sharp knife, slice each chicken breast into four pieces and divide these pieces between the four plates, together with the walnuts. Serve immediately.

TIP Blueberries are loaded with fiber, which will keep you feeling full for longer, and provide you with almost 25 percent of your daily value of vitamin C.

AVOCADO CHICKEN SALAD

This salad is great for a busy midweek supper as it only takes minutes to prepare.

386 CALORIES | 20G FAT | 3.5G SATURATES | 12G CARBS | 10G SUGAR | 0.2G SALT | 39G PROTEIN | 4G FIBER

SERVES 4

4 skinless chicken breasts

1 tablespoon olive oil

1 large ripe avocado, peeled and pitted (or 2 smaller avocados)

a squeeze of lime

1 green apple, chopped into small cubes

½ cup red seedless grapes, halved

2 tablespoons chopped walnuts

2 tablespoons dried cranberries or raisins

a handful of cilantro, finely chopped

juice of 1 lime

sea salt

2 little gem lettuces or 1 head of romaine, leaves separated

1. Turn on the broiler. Rub the chicken all over with a little olive oil and broil for 4 to 5 minutes on each side until lightly charred and cooked through.

2. Place the avocado in a large bowl and mash to a chunky/ creamy consistency with a squeeze of lime.

3. Place the apple, grapes, walnuts, cranberries or raisins, and cilantro in a bowl, and toss to combine. Add the lime juice and the salt to taste and toss again.

4. Place a few lettuce leaves on each plate and spoon over the fruit and nut mix. Serve with the chicken (sliced if you prefer) and a large spoonful of creamy avocado on the side.

TIP To keep this salad from turning brown, try leaving the stone from the avocado in the mixture until ready to serve. And if you'd like something with a more mayo-like consistency, try the avocado mayo recipe on page 48.

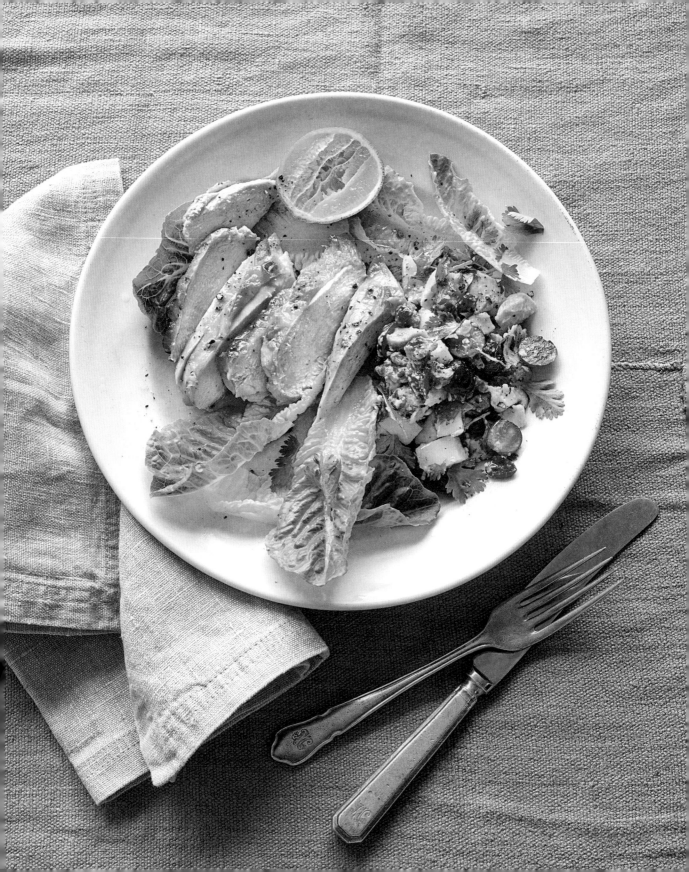

CHICKEN LIVER SALAD
WITH FRIED ONIONS

This dish is deservedly a classic of French cuisine and makes a fantastically simple mid-week supper. Chicken liver also couldn't be better for you—it's inexpensive, full of protein and really delicious. The trick is to fry it in a hot pan for just a couple of minutes on each side. Don't overcook it!

174 CALORIES | 8.5G FAT | 1.5G SATURATES | 3G CARBS | 2.5G SUGAR | 0.4G SALT | 20G PROTEIN | 2.5G FIBER

SERVES 4

2 tablespoons olive oil

1 red onion, finely sliced

14 ounces chicken livers

7 ounces (about 5 cups) fresh spinach

3½ ounces (about 3 cups) watercress

1 teaspoon balsamic vinegar

English mustard, to serve

1. Heat 1 tablespoon of oil in a large non-stick sauté pan over medium-high heat and fry the onion for 3 to 4 minutes until nicely browned. Transfer to a plate and set aside.

2. Turn the heat up to high, add ½ tablespoon olive oil to the pan, and cook the chicken livers for 2 minutes on each side until they are a lovely nutty brown on the outside and pink and tender in the middle. Transfer to a plate and set aside.

3. In a large bowl, mix together the spinach and watercress, and toss with remaining olive oil and a little balsamic vinegar.

4. Divide the dressed salad leaves between four plates, arrange the chicken livers on top, and sprinkle with the red onion. Drizzle any remaining juice from the pan over the meat and serve with a spoonful of English mustard.

TIP This dish is an iron-rich feast as the liver, watercress, and spinach all contain huge amounts of this essential mineral—great for times when you feel weak, tired, and especially run down.

GRILLED CHICKEN SALAD
WITH ROASTED TOMATOES & POACHED EGG

I just love this protein-rich salad. It's so easy to make and yet so satisfying, plus the roasted tomatoes add a really delicious sweetness that complements the chicken and egg perfectly.

456 CALORIES | 32G FAT | 5.5G SATURATES | 4G CARBS | 3.5G SUGAR | 0.9G SALT | 37G PROTEIN | 1.7G FIBER

SERVES 4

for the marinade and dressing

¼ cup sherry vinegar or champagne vinegar

1 tablespoon Dijon mustard

1 tablespoon white truffle oil

1 teaspoon chopped fresh thyme leaves

2 garlic cloves, finely chopped

½ teaspoon sea salt

¼ teaspoon freshly ground black pepper

½ cup extra virgin olive oil

for the salad

4 × 4-ounce boneless skinless chicken breast halves

2 cups cherry tomatoes, halved

4 eggs

2 teaspoons vinegar (any kind)

7 ounces (about 5 cups) salad greens (a mix of butter lettuce, frisée, baby spinach, etc.)

1. Preheat the oven to 425°F.

2. In a small bowl, combine the vinegar, mustard, truffle oil, thyme, garlic, and salt and pepper, then slowly whisk in the extra virgin olive oil. Pour about half of the mixture into a large resealable plastic bag, and reserve the rest. Place the chicken in the marinade, seal the bag and turn to coat the meat thoroughly, then refrigerate for at least 1 hour or overnight.

3. In a large bowl, toss the tomatoes in 2 tablespoons of the reserved dressing, then spread them out over a baking sheet, and roast in the oven for 15 to 20 minutes until slightly shriveled. Set aside to cool.

4. Remove the chicken from the bag and drain and discard the marinade. Place a grill pan over high heat and cook the chicken for 4 to 7 minutes on each side or until cooked through. Set aside to cool slightly, then slice at a diagonal.

5. Meanwhile, bring a saucepan of water to a simmer. Add the vinegar and slide in each freshly cracked egg. Poach for about 3 minutes or to your desired doneness, then remove with a slotted spoon, place briefly in cold water to remove any vinegar and drain on paper towels.

6. In a large bowl, combine the salad greens with the remaining dressing and toss to coat. Divide between four serving plates, top with the roasted tomatoes and sliced chicken, and finish with a freshly poached egg.

GRILLED SALMON SALAD

Orange and salmon are a lovely combination in this simple, fresh, and zesty salad.

794 CALORIES | 60G FAT | 9G SATURATES | 23G CARBS | 22G SUGAR | 1.7G SALT | 37G PROTEIN | 9G FIBER

SERVES 2

for the orange vinaigrette

½ large orange

2 teaspoons finely chopped shallots

1 teaspoon raw honey

1 teaspoon seasoned rice vinegar

¼ cup sunflower oil

1 teaspoon extra virgin olive oil

sea salt and freshly ground black pepper

¼ teaspoon orange oil (optional, see Tip)

10 asparagus spears, trimmed

2 × 5-ounce salmon fillets

4 teaspoons olive oil

sea salt and freshly ground black pepper

4 ounces (about 2 cups) salad leaves

⅔ cup pitted Kalamata olives, halved

1 orange, peeled and segmented

½ red onion, thinly sliced

1. First make the vinaigrette: Zest the orange and squeeze the juice into a small bowl. Add the zest, shallots, honey, and rice vinegar to the orange juice and whisk together. Next add the sunflower oil and olive oil slowly, in a steady stream, while constantly whisking. Add the salt, pepper, and orange oil and whisk again until combined.

2. Turn on the broiler. Bring a saucepan of water to a boil and cook the asparagus for 30 seconds, then drain and place under cold running water to stop the cooking process, and set aside.

3. Rub the salmon fillets all over with half the olive oil and season lightly. Place under the broiler for 5 to 10 minutes on each side, or until done to your liking. Set aside.

4. Place the salad leaves, olives, orange, onion, and half of the vinaigrette in a large bowl and toss to combine.

5. Toss the asparagus in the remaining oil and season lightly, then place under the hot grill for about 3 minutes until lightly charred.

6. Divide the salad between two plates, place the asparagus and salmon on top, and drizzle the remaining dressing over the salmon. Serve immediately.

TIP Boyajian Orange Oil is available at specialty food stores. It is very strong so only a small amount is needed.

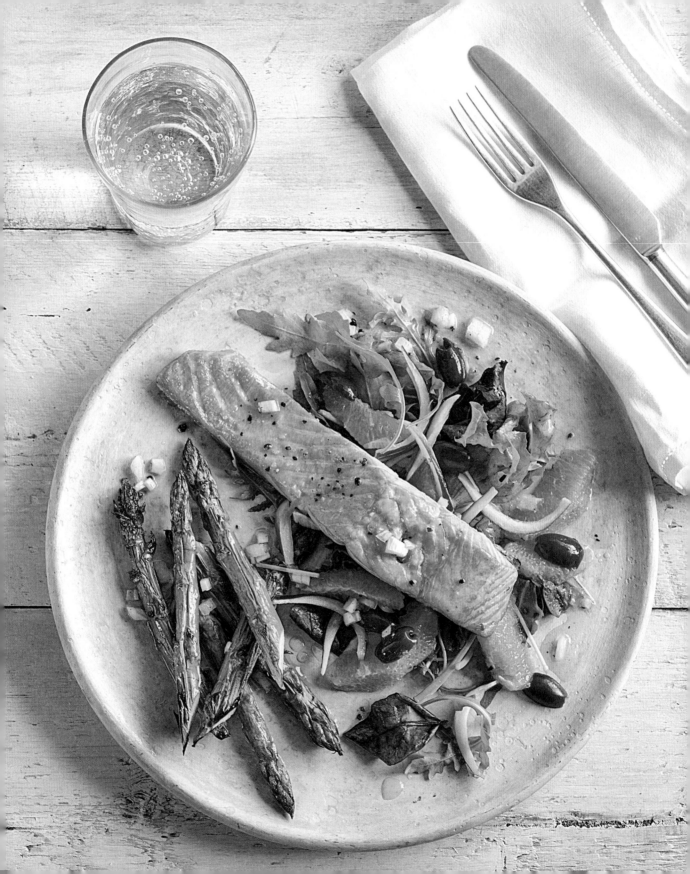

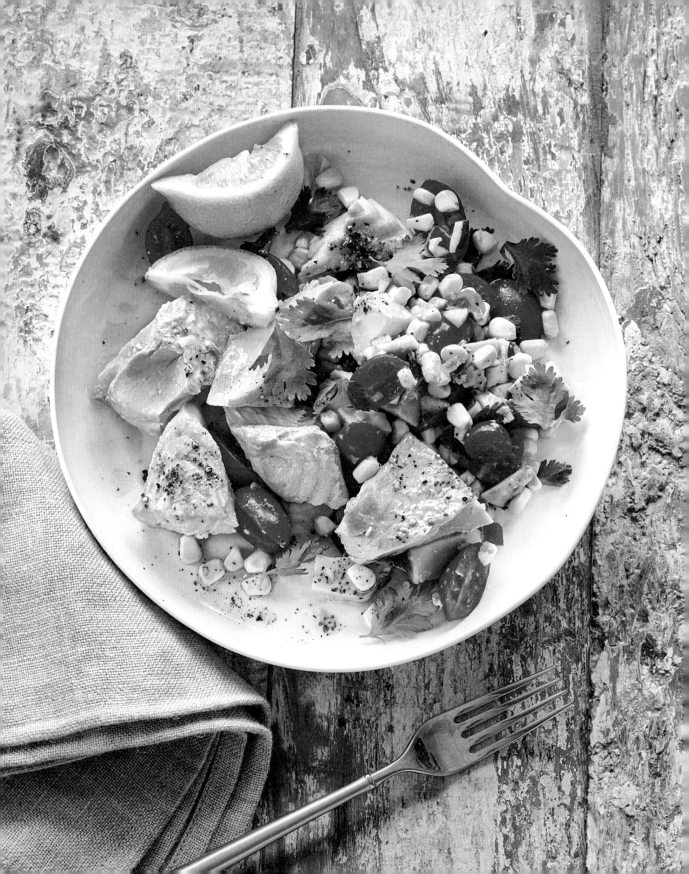

SALMON, CORN & AVOCADO SALAD

I love the textures in this salad. Try and use the freshest corn you can find as then there is no need to cook it and it's deliciously sweet and crunchy.

590 CALORIES | 43G FAT | 7.5G SATURATES | 11G CARBS | 4G SUGAR | 0.2G SALT | 37G PROTEIN | 4.5G FIBER

SERVES 4

for the salad

4 ears fresh corn, kernels removed from cob

10 cherry tomatoes, halved

1 small avocado, peeled, pitted, and diced

½ red onion, finely chopped

a large handful of fresh cilantro, finely chopped

2 tablespoons extra virgin olive oil

2 tablespoons champagne vinegar

2 tablespoons red wine vinegar

for the salmon

4 × 5½-ounce boneless, skinless salmon fillets

½ tablespoon extra virgin olive oil

sea salt and freshly ground black pepper

½ lemon

1. Turn on the broiler.

2. Place the corn, tomatoes, avocado, onion, cilantro, oil, and vinegars in a large bowl and toss gently to combine. Set aside.

3. Lightly brush each salmon fillet all over with a little olive oil and season to taste. Place the fillets under the broiler and cook for about 4 to 5 minutes on each side.

4. Fork the cooked salmon into small chunks so you can see the juicy pink flesh and squeeze over a little lemon.

5. Divide the salad between four serving bowls, lay the salmon on top, and serve immediately while the fish is still warm.

VENISON & POMEGRANATE SALAD

Venison is a very lean meat so is excellent if you're watching your weight. It's best served on the rare side so make sure you only cook with very fresh meat.

285 CALORIES | 6G FAT | 2G SATURATES | 20G CARBS | 19G SUGAR | 0.8G SALT | 36G PROTEIN | 4G FIBER

SERVES 4

a drizzle of olive oil

sea salt and freshly ground black pepper

2 × 10½-ounce venison steaks

¾ pound (about 10 cups) mixed salad leaves

½ red onion, finely sliced

1 orange, peeled and sliced into segments

1 cup pomegranate seeds

for the balsamic vinaigrette

¼ cup plus 2 tablespoons balsamic vinegar

juice of ½ large lemon

2 tablespoons Dijon mustard

1 garlic clove, crushed

1 teaspoon dried basil

1 tablespoon maple syrup

1. Drizzle a little oil into a large non-stick frying pan, lightly season the venison, and then sear over high heat for about 3 minutes on each side. Turn off the heat and let the meat rest in the pan for 5 minutes, then turn and let it rest for another few minutes.

2. Meanwhile, make the dressing. Place all the ingredients in a jar and shake well.

3. Place the salad leaves in a large bowl and toss together with a little dressing. Divide the salad between four plates, add the red onion and orange segments, and sprinkle over the pomegranate seeds.

4. Place the rested meat on a cutting board and, with a sharp knife, slice the steaks thinly. Arrange the slices over the salad and serve immediately.

TIP Venison is a great healthy eating choice—it has more protein than any other red meat and contains even more iron than beef, so is good for energy levels. Also, because of all the wild and pasture food that deer graze on, the small amount of fat in venison is generally high in conjugated linoleic acid, which is thought to protect against heart disease and cancer.

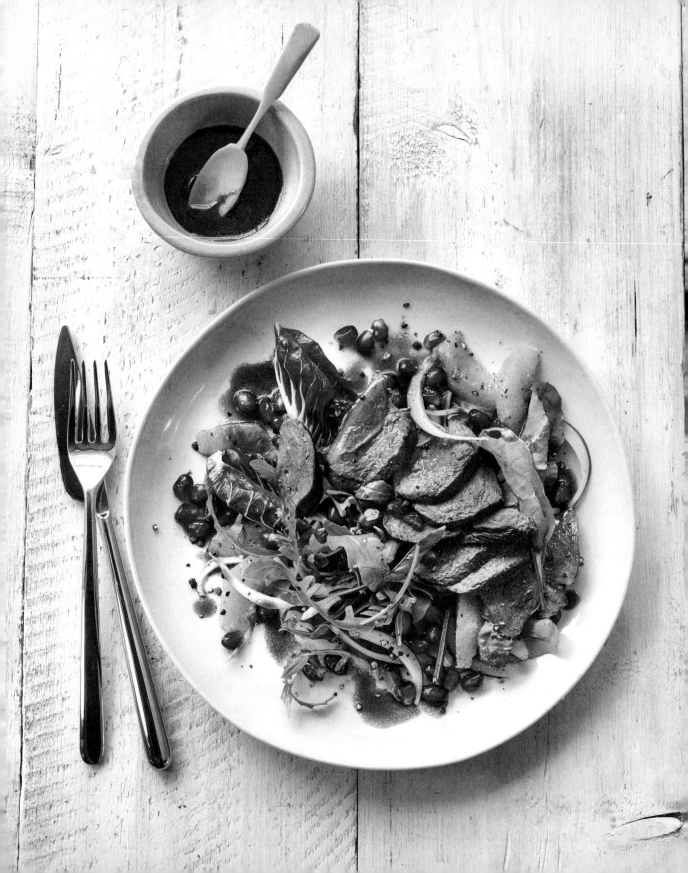

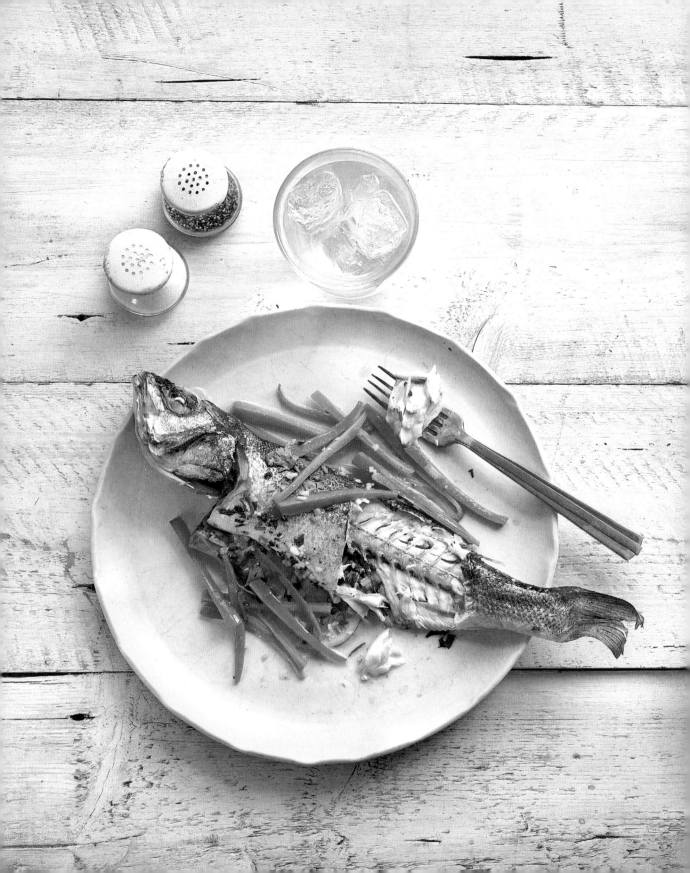

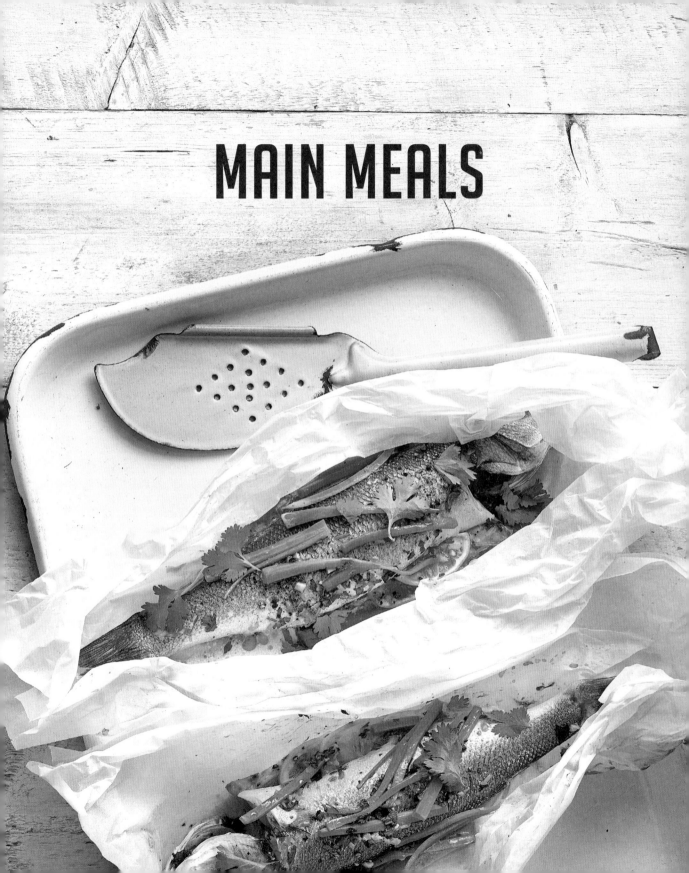

MAIN MEALS

BUTTERNUT SQUASH CURRY

I try not to cook with large amounts of butternut squash as it's quite high in carbs. However, as there's no protein added to this curry, you'll need the carbs to fill you up, plus I love the way the squash and coconut milk cook down and flavor each other—it's a true Thai classic.

269 CALORIES | 15G FAT | 7G SATURATES | 22G CARBS | 14G SUGAR | 0.3G SALT | 7G PROTEIN | 8G FIBER

SERVES 4

1 medium butternut squash, peeled, seeded and chopped into 2-inch pieces

2 tablespoons olive oil

1 small yellow onion, finely chopped

4 zucchini, sliced lengthways, then quartered

2 teaspoons Thai red curry paste

1-inch piece fresh ginger, grated

1 × 13.5-ounce can light coconut milk

7 ounces (about 5 cups) fresh spinach

a handful of fresh cilantro, finely chopped

1. Preheat the oven to 400°F.

2. Place the butternut squash in a roasting pan, drizzle with a tablespoon of oil, and toss to coat, then roast in the oven for 30 minutes.

3. Heat the remaining olive oil in a large saucepan over high heat and cook the onion for 2 minutes until translucent. Add the zucchini and cook for an additional 3 minutes, then lower the heat to medium, add the butternut squash, stir together and cook for a few more minutes.

4. Add the curry paste and ginger and stir to coat, then add the coconut milk and cook, covered, for 5 minutes.

5. Add the spinach, stir and cook for an additional few minutes, then garnish with a sprinkling of cilantro and serve immediately.

TIP Ginger is a great spice to cook with as it boosts the metabolism and has been shown to increase thermogenesis in the body, where your body burns stored fat to create heat. Research shows that it can boost your metabolism by up to 5 percent, and increase fat burning by up to 16 percent.

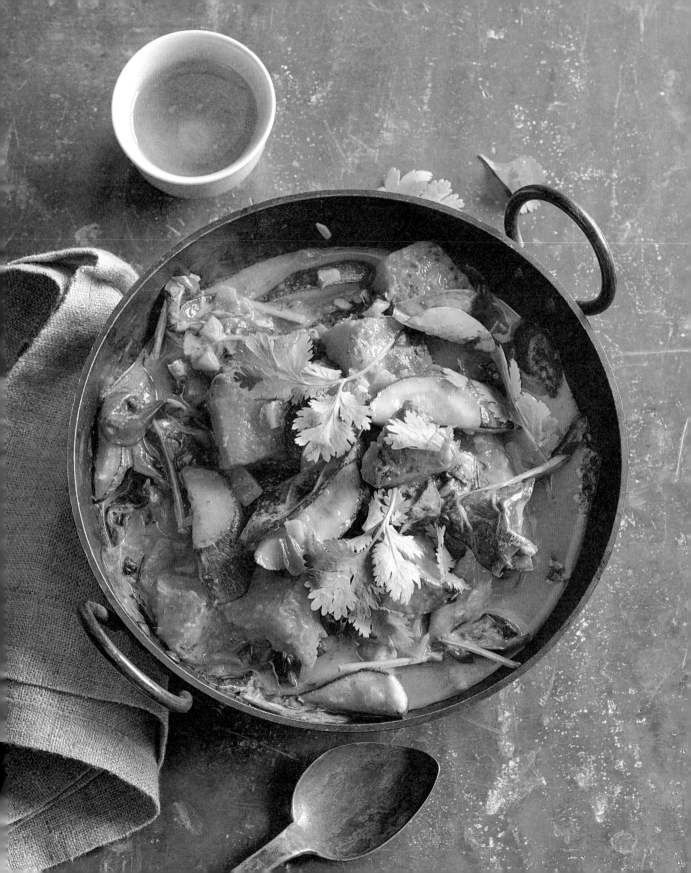

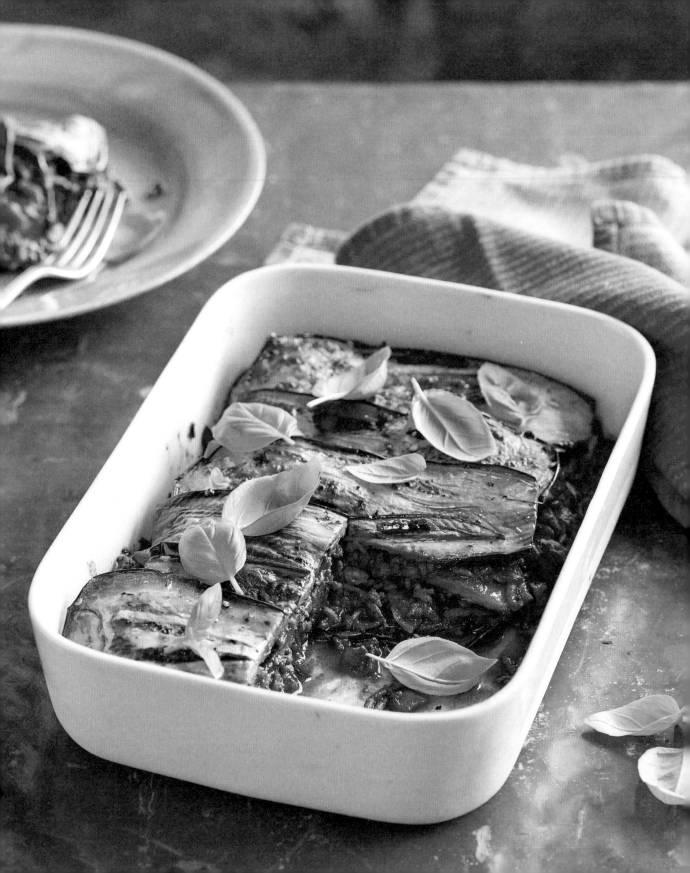

EGGPLANT LASAGNE

This is a delicious, healthy pasta-free lasagne. You can layer the eggplant or roll it up like cannelloni and either way is perfect for a satisfying Italian-style feast.

318 CALORIES | 20G FAT | 7G SATURATES | 8G CARBS | 7G SUGAR | 0.1G SALT | 24G PROTEIN | 7G FIBER

SERVES 4

2 tablespoons olive oil

2 large eggplant, cut into ¼-inch slices

½ yellow onion, finely chopped

1 pound lean ground beef

2 garlic cloves, crushed

1 tablespoon sun-dried tomato paste

2 tablespoons tomato paste

a handful of fresh basil, shredded

2 tablespoons vegetable stock

5 ounces (about 4 cups) salad leaves, to serve

1. Preheat the oven to 350°F.

2. Heat 1 tablespoon of olive oil in a large non-stick grill pan over high heat and grill the eggplant slices for a couple of minutes on each side until nice and brown (you may have to do this in batches as it's important not to crowd the pan).

3. Heat the remaining olive oil in a large sauté pan and cook the onion over medium to high heat for 2 to 3 minutes.

4. Add the ground beef and sauté for 2 to 3 minutes to brown, then add the garlic, tomato pastes, a tablespoon of basil, and the stock. Cover and simmer for 3 to 4 minutes.

5. Take a baking dish and line the base with eggplant slices. Spoon over a third of the meat sauce, then cover with a layer of eggplant slices. Repeat until all the sauce is used up, finishing with a layer of eggplant on top.

6. Cover with foil and place in the oven for 15 to 18 minutes. If you prefer a crunchy top, remove the foil at the end, spray with a little extra oil, and place under the broiler for 2 to 3 minutes.

7. Serve with a sprinkling of fresh basil and a bright, fresh green salad.

DINNER FOR A KING

This is the dinner I cook when I want to indulge myself and my family and friends.
I often add lobster if it's a special occasion or swap the canned crab for fresh, and
scallops make a great addition too.

486 CALORIES | 29G FAT | 7G SATURATES | 2.5G CARBS | 2G SUGAR | 6G SALT | 52G PROTEIN | 3G FIBER

- -

SERVES 4

4 to 6 shallots, finely chopped

1 tablespoon chopped
    fresh dill

7 ounces canned white
    crab meat

7 ounces (about 5 cups)
    arugula

1.3 pounds Scottish smoked
    salmon

1 avocado, peeled, pitted,
    and sliced

2 hard-boiled eggs, quartered

3 tablespoons salmon caviar
    (roe)

sea salt and freshly ground
    black pepper

1 lemon, quartered

1. In a small mixing bowl, toss together the
   shallots, dill, and crab meat and set aside.

2. Divide the arugula between four serving plates
   and top with the smoked salmon, avocado, and
   two egg quarters, then spoon over the salmon
   caviar.

3. Add the crab meat mixture to the plate, season
   to taste, and finish with a squeeze of lemon.
   Serve immediately.

- -

TIP Fish eggs (also known as roe) are generally associated
with a fancy caviar canapé and are therefore very
overlooked as a kitchen ingredient, which is a shame as they
don't need to cost the earth (especially salmon or carp roe),
plus they're full of micro-nutrients and omega-3 fatty acids
and, most importantly, they're very tasty. The best way to
ensure quality is to buy fresh from your local fishmonger.
Roe in a jar or a can is often full of preservatives so read
the label carefully.

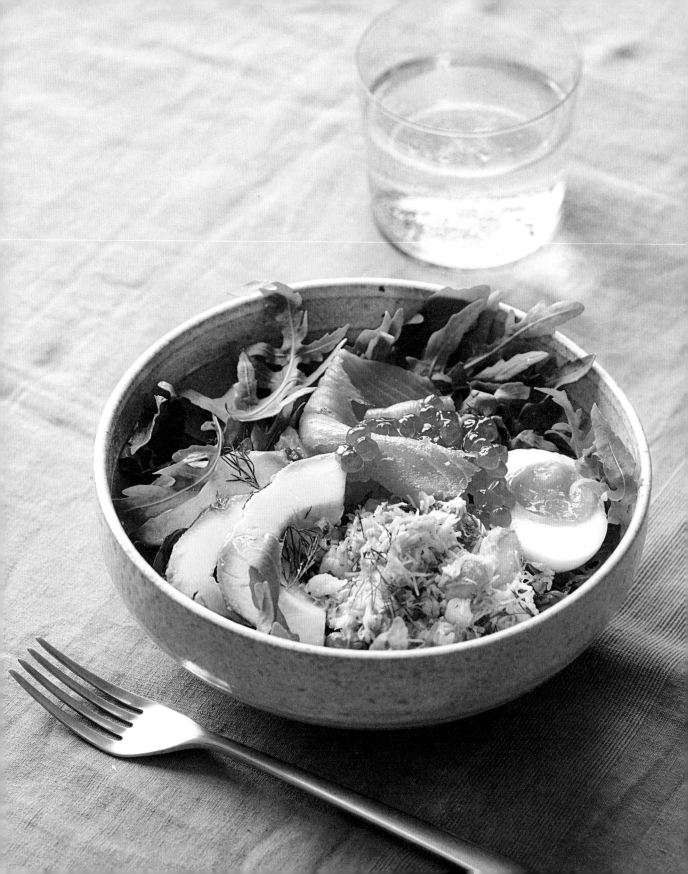

STUFFED SQUID
WITH SHRIMP

This recipe works well with both large and baby squid, although the former are quite a bit easier to fill!

565 CALORIES | 26G FAT | 5G SATURATES | 4G CARBS | 4G SUGAR | 2.6G SALT | 78G PROTEIN | 1G FIBER

SERVES 4

2.2 pounds fresh squid, cleaned

1 pound skinless salmon fillet

12 ounces shelled raw shrimp, (large if possible)

juice of ½ lemon

1 egg

1 tablespoon coconut aminos

1 garlic clove, crushed

a handful of fresh cilantro

freshly ground black pepper

1 × 14.5-ounce can chopped tomatoes

⅔ cup vegetable or fish stock

1 tablespoon olive oil

1. First prepare the squid: Remove the tentacles and reserve. Pull away the wings, remove the head, and empty the main tube of cartilage and slime. Pull or cut away the eyes and beak, and remove anything else that feels hard or slimy from the tentacles. Discard everything but the cleaned tentacles and main body tube. Wash well and dry.

2. To make the filling, place the salmon, shrimp, lemon juice, egg, coconut aminos, garlic, and cilantro in a blender and purée until smooth.

3. Stuff each piece of squid with the filling to about two-thirds full and secure the end with a wooden cocktail stick. Season with black pepper and reserve until ready to cook.

4. Place the tomatoes and stock in a wide, deep sauté pan over medium heat and bring to a low simmer, stirring to combine.

5. Heat the oil in another non-stick pan over moderate heat and cook the squid for 2 minutes on each side.

6. Transfer the squid to the pan with the tomato sauce and cook, covered, over medium to low heat for about 12 to 15 minutes. Turn half way through cooking time.

7. Serve the squid with a ladleful of tomato sauce and some extra cilantro sprinkled on top.

GARLIC SHRIMP
WITH BOK CHOY

For this dish, the bigger the shrimp the better. Tiger shrimp from Southeast Asia are the largest and in my opinion the best-tasting.

228 CALORIES | 4.5G FAT | 0.8G SATURATES | 3.5G CARBS | 2G SUGAR | 1.6G SALT | 42G PROTEIN | 3G FIBER

SERVES 4

2 pounds large raw tiger shrimp

1 tablespoon olive oil

juice of ½ lemon

4 garlic cloves, finely chopped

1 tablespoon coconut aminos

6 heads bok choy, leaves separated

a handful of flat-leaf parsley, finely chopped

1. Keep the head on each shrimp but peel the body and devein it by slicing through the back. Take out the dark lining and discard it.

2. Spray a large non-stick sauté pan with a little olive oil, place on high heat, and cook the shrimp for 2 to 3 minutes on each side, depending on how big they are.

3. Add the lemon juice, 2 garlic cloves, and soy sauce, then take off the heat and stir fry for 1 minute while the pan is still hot. Leave to stand.

4. In another pan, heat 1 tablespoon olive oil and, when hot, stir-fry the bok choy for about 3 to 5 minutes. Add the remaining garlic, then cook for an additional minute.

5. Serve the shrimp with the bok choy, a sprinkling of parsley, and a fresh squeeze of lemon.

TIP I recommend you keep the heads of the shrimp on for cooking as there is so much flavor there. You can eat them too if you like—they are tasty—but it's up to you!

PAD THAI

This is the closest you can get to the flavors of a pad thai on the Paleo diet—true comfort food at its best!

129 CALORIES | 5G FAT | 1G SATURATES | 6G CARBS | 4G SUGAR | 0.8G SALT | 14G PROTEIN | 3G FIBER

SERVES 4

for the marinade
1 teaspoon fish sauce
juice of ½ lemon
1 teaspoon chile powder
1 teaspoon maple syrup

olive oil spray, for cooking
3 zucchini, sliced into matchsticks
a large handful of cilantro leaves, finely chopped
2 scallions, finely chopped
1 cup bean sprouts
12 tiger shrimp, peeled and deveined (see page 109)
2 tablespoons cashews, to garnish

1. First make the marinade: In a large bowl, mix together the fish sauce, lemon juice, chile powder, and maple syrup and set aside.

2. Heat a large non-stick wok over high heat, spray with olive oil and sauté the zucchini for 2 minutes.

3. Remove the zucchini from the pan and add to the marinade. Stir to mix, then add the cilantro, scallions and bean sprouts.

4. Meanwhile, spray the wok again with a little oil and sauté the shrimp for 2 minutes on each side until cooked through.

5. Divide the vegetables between four serving plates and distribute the shrimp on top. Garnish with the cashews and serve.

TIP Fish sauce is made from fermenting tiny fish, such as anchovies, in brine and then preserving the liquid, so it should contain only two Paleo-friendly ingredients—fish and salt. However, check the labels and avoid any products with unnecessary extras such as hydrolyzed wheat protein and fructose! Red Boat Fish Sauce is a good brand to look for.

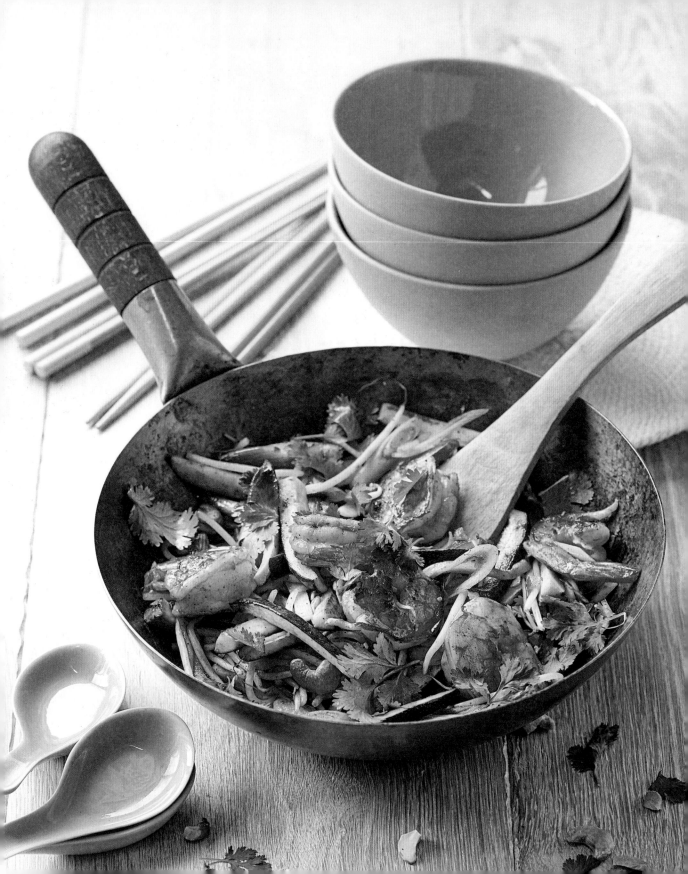

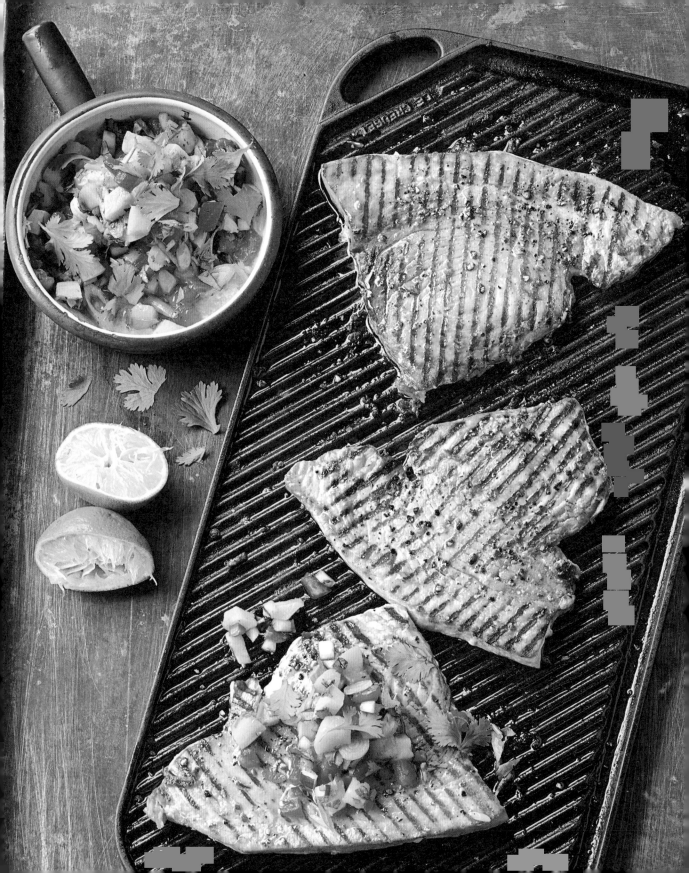

GRILLED SWORDFISH
WITH MANGO SALSA

Swordfish is a lovely meaty fish that holds up really well to high heat so is the perfect choice for a barbecue. Try this dish with tuna and salmon as an alternative too.

326 CALORIES | 12G FAT | 2.5G SATURATES | 11G CARBS | 11G SUGAR | 0.7G SALT | 42G PROTEIN | 4G FIBER

SERVES 4

for the salsa

½ ripe mango, peeled, pitted, and finely diced

1 small red chile, finely diced

4 plum tomatoes, seeded and finely diced

½ red onion, finely chopped

3 scallions, finely sliced

2 garlic cloves, finely chopped

a handful of fresh cilantro, chopped

juice of 1 lemon or lime

5 ounces (about 4 cups) salad leaves

4 × 7½-ounce swordfish steaks (about ¾ inch thick)

sea salt and freshly ground black pepper

1 tablespoon olive oil

5 ounces (about 4 cups) salad leaves, to serve

1. First make the salsa: Place all the ingredients in a large bowl, mix to combine thoroughly, and season to taste.

2. Lightly season the swordfish on both sides. Heat the oil in a grill pan until really hot and cook the steaks for 2 minutes on each side, then cover, take off the heat and keep in the hot pan for 3 to 4 minutes.

3. Arrange the salsa on a plate, top with the fish, and serve with a side salad of mixed leaves.

TIP Cooking swordfish is easy. The trick is to ensure the grill pan is nice and hot before you start and to cook it all the way through to the point where the texture is a little flaky but not mushy.

SESAME TUNA STEAK
WITH WOK-FRIED VEGETABLES

Sesame with tuna is one of those classic flavor combinations that I turn to again and again. I love sesame oil too but it has such a strong, distinctive flavor that a little goes a long way.

453 CALORIES | 23G FAT | 4G SATURATES | 4.5G CARBS | 4G SUGAR | 0.5G SALT | 53G PROTEIN | 6G FIBER

- -

SERVES 4

6 tablespoons sesame seeds

4 × 6-ounce tuna steaks

2 tablespoons olive oil

½ large yellow onion, thinly sliced

8 asparagus, trimmed and sliced into 2-inch pieces

7 ounces (about 5 cups) fresh spinach

juice of ½ lemon

1 small red bird's-eye chile, very finely chopped (retain the seeds for extra heat)

1 tablespoon sesame oil

sea salt and freshly ground black pepper

4 scallions, finely sliced

a handful of fresh cilantro

1. Spread the sesame seeds out over a large plate and then, one at a time, press both sides of the tuna steaks down firmly onto the plate so the seeds stick on all sides.

2. Heat 1 tablespoon oil in a large non-stick frying pan and, when hot, sear the tuna steaks for 1 to 2 minutes on each side. Take the tuna out of the pan and set aside.

3. Heat the remaining oil in a large wok and cook the onions for 2 minutes, then add the asparagus and stir-fry for an additional few minutes.

4. Now add the spinach and stir until it wilts, then add the lemon juice and take off the heat.

5. Add the chile and sesame oil and mix well, then season to taste.

6. Divide the wok-fried vegetables between four serving plates. Arrange the tuna on top and sprinkle with scallions and cilantro to garnish.

- -

TIP Nothing is worse than overcooked tuna. It's such a waste of good quality and fairly expensive fish so I always recommend you keep it rare on the inside.

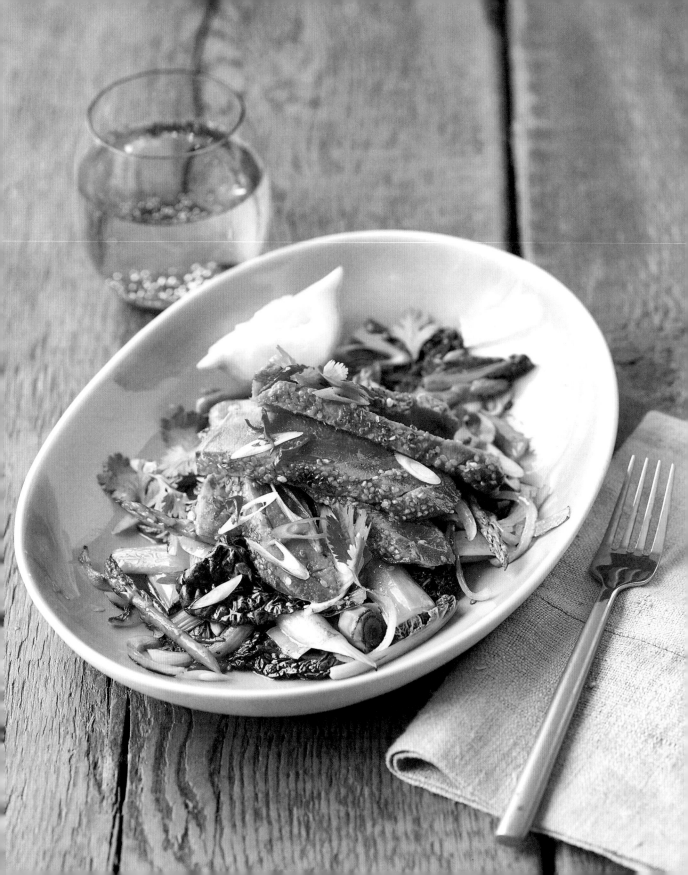

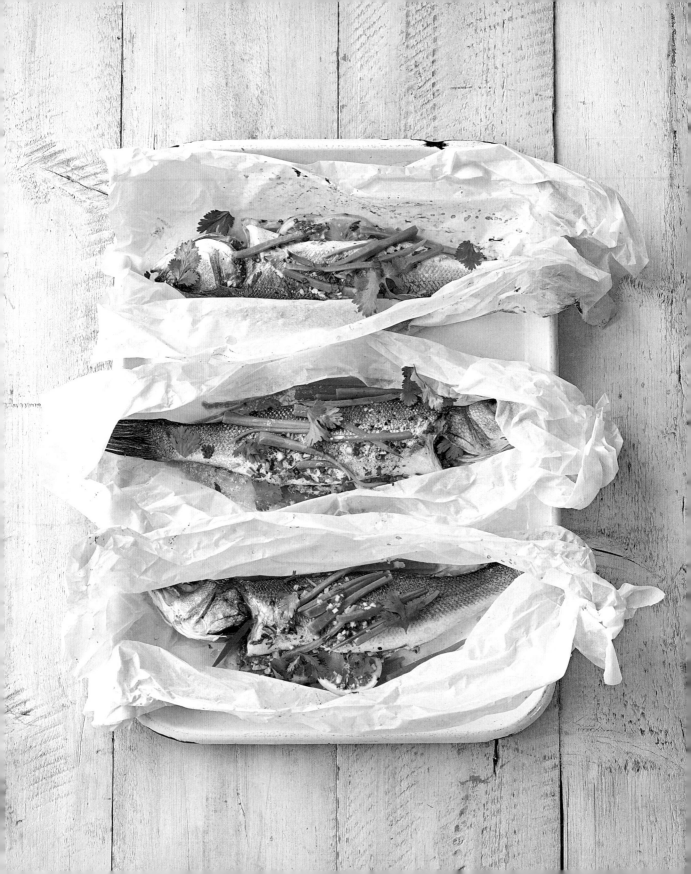

SEA BASS PARCELS

Filling the cavity of a fish with herbs and spices beautifully infuses the flesh with flavor, plus wrapping it up keeps it nice and moist.

445 CALORIES | 22G FAT | 5.5G SATURATES | 12G CARBS | 11G SUGAR | 1G SALT | 45G PROTEIN | 8G FIBER

SERVES 4

1 large handful of fresh cilantro

1 garlic clove, peeled

1-inch piece fresh ginger, grated

½ small red bird's-eye chile

4 whole sea bass, gutted, cleaned, and scaled

1 cup fish stock

3½ tablespoons light coconut milk

4 large carrots, peeled and sliced into matchsticks

2 lemons, 1 thinly sliced, 1 quartered

1.3 pounds asparagus, trimmed

freshly ground black pepper

squeeze of lemon juice

1. Preheat the oven 350°F.

2. Place the cilantro, garlic, ginger, and chile in a food processor and process until finely chopped.

3. Rinse out the cavity of each fish under cold running water to ensure it is completely clean and check all the scales have been removed. (You can use the back of a knife to do this, running it in the opposite direction to the scales.)

4. Spread a quarter of the spice mix inside the cavity of each fish and place each one on a piece of lightly oiled foil or baking parchment that has been twisted to form a shallow bowl shape.

5. Mix together the stock and coconut milk and pour over the fish in each foil packet. Add some carrot sticks and a few slices of lemon and cover with another sheet of foil and seal together. Cook in the oven for 20 to 25 minutes.

6. Meanwhile, place a large grill pan over a high heat and grill the asparagus on all sides until nicely charred. Season with a twist of pepper, dress with a squeeze of lemon, and keep warm.

7. Check that the fish is cooked through: the flesh should be firm and flake easily, then serve with the grilled asparagus and lemon quarters, and don't forget to spoon the juices from the parcel over the top.

SEAWEED SALMON

The beauty of this dish is that the seaweed protects the fish while cooking so keeps it beautifully moist. Seaweed is of course a great accompaniment to almost any fish so try this recipe with trout, cod, sea bass, or whatever you happen to have to hand.

475 CALORIES | 33G FAT | 6G SATURATES | 0.5G CARBS | 0.5G SUGAR | 0.3G SALT | 42G PROTEIN | 2G FIBER

SERVES 4

for the marinade

1-inch piece fresh ginger, grated

juice of ½ lime

a handful of fresh cilantro, finely chopped

1 garlic clove, crushed

1 teaspoon sesame oil

1 small red bird's-eye chile, finely chopped

for the salmon parcels

8 nori (seaweed) sheets

1 teaspoon wasabi paste (optional)

4 × 7-ounce skinless salmon fillets

for the bok choy

1 tablespoon olive oil

2 heads bok choy

2 garlic cloves, finely chopped

1. First make the marinade: In a small bowl, mix together the ginger, lime, cilantro, garlic, sesame oil, and chile, then set aside.

2. Lay out four sheets of seaweed paper on a chopping board. If you are using the wasabi, take a chopstick or knife and run a thin line of paste across each sheet, then lay the salmon on top. Drizzle the marinade over each salmon fillet, then lay a seaweed sheet on top and rest for 2 minutes so the seaweed absorbs the liquid and the flavors. Now fold over all the edges to make a parcel.

3. Place the salmon parcels in a bamboo steamer and steam for 12 to 15 minutes.

4. Meanwhile, place the oil in a wok over high heat, separate the bok choy leaves and stir-fry with the garlic for a few minutes until wilted.

5. Transfer the salmon to a chopping board and, with a sharp knife, slice each parcel into three or four pieces. Serve with the bok choy on the side.

TIP Wasabi is a Japanese plant in the same family as horseradish, cabbage, and mustard. In its completely natural form, it is a Paleo ingredient and yet, sadly, as it's a plant that's hard to grow, the "wasabi" condiment you're most likely served at sushi restaurants is not wasabi at all. If it is green, it has food coloring in it, and it might also contain some form of starch too. You should be able to find powdered wasabi root at Japanese markets, but be warned that it will be pricey!

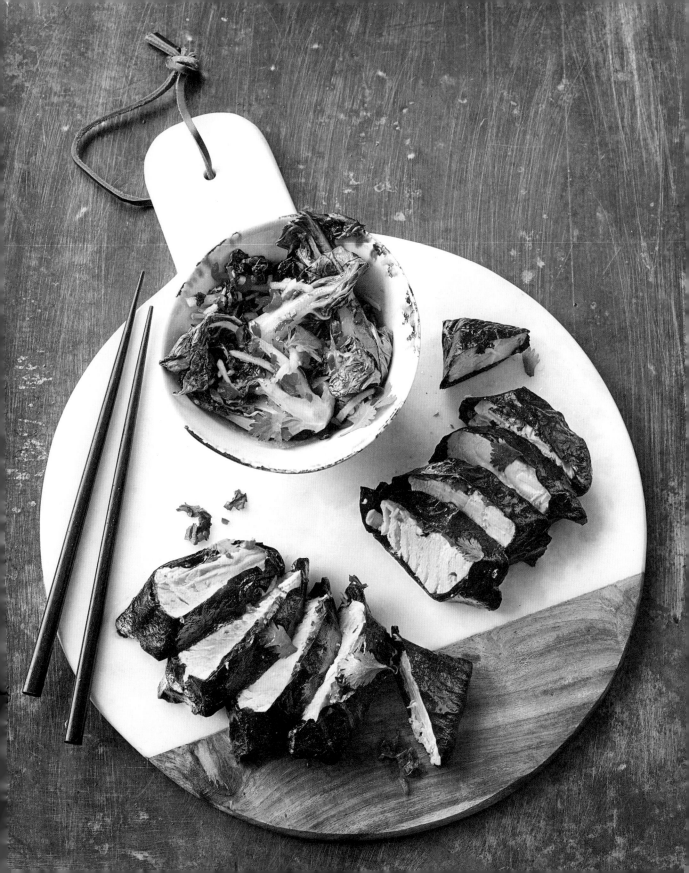

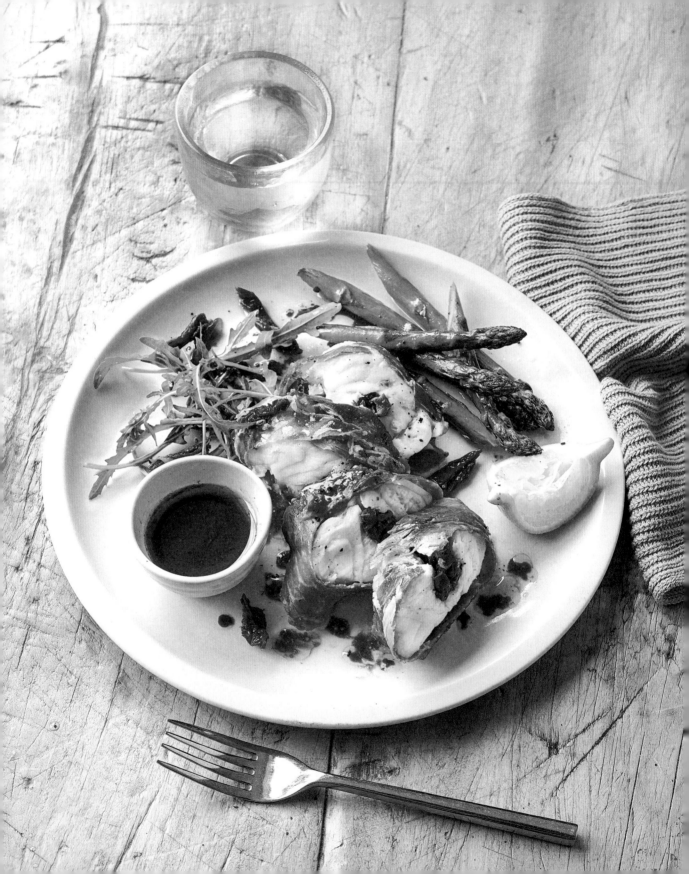

ROASTED MONKFISH
WRAPPED IN PROSCIUTTO

Wrapping fish in prosciutto and then roasting it in the oven is such a simple but fail-safe way of achieving really wonderful flavor. Try it with cod, haddock, salmon, and chicken. It's always delicious!

573 CALORIES | 29G FAT | 5G SATURATES | 5G CARBS | 4G SUGAR | 3G SALT | 72G PROTEIN | 4G FIBER

SERVES 4

4 × 12-ounce monkfish tails

1 cup sun-dried tomatoes in olive oil

12 slices prosciutto or Parma ham

14 ounces (about 10 cups) arugula

¾ pound asparagus, ends trimmed

1 tablespoon olive oil

for the dressing

4 tablespoons olive oil.

2 tablespoons balsamic vinegar

1 tablespoon Dijon mustard

juice of 1 lemon

1. Preheat the oven to 400°F.

2. Place the monkfish tails on a chopping board and, using a sharp knife, make a 1-inch deep incision down the length of the tail.

3. Drain the sun-dried tomatoes on a paper towel to absorb the excess oil, then slice into thin strips, and then tuck these slices into the incision you've just made down the length of the fish.

4. Wrap the monkfish with prosciutto so that all the flesh is covered and place on a foil-lined roasting pan. Roast in the oven for 20 to 25 minutes or until completely cooked through.

5. Meanwhile, whisk all the salad dressing ingredients in a small bowl and then toss over the arugula.

6. Heat a large grill pan over medium-high heat and grill the asparagus spears on all sides until nicely marked. As soon as they're done, dress them with a squeeze of lemon.

7. Serve the fish alongside the asparagus and salad with a few additional sun-dried tomatoes if you would like.

SEARED SCALLOPS ON PARSNIP PURÉE

If you reduce the portion size, this makes a great dinner party starter, or even serve on Chinese porcelain spoons as a canapé. As a main course, I recommend you serve this with some wilted spinach on the side.

504 CALORIES | 16G FAT | 3G SATURATES | 26G CARBS | 11G SUGAR | 1G SALT | 56G PROTEIN | 10G FIBER

SERVES 4

1 whole garlic bulb, halved

4 to 6 tablespoons olive oil

4 to 6 large parsnips, peeled and quartered

sea salt and freshly ground black pepper

2 pounds scallops (find the largest you can)

a handful of fresh chives

1. Preheat the oven to 425°F.

2. Place the garlic bulb halves in a small ovenproof dish and drizzle with olive oil, then wrap in foil, and bake in the oven for 30 minutes. Set aside to cool, then squeeze the roasted garlic flesh out of the skin.

3. Bring a pan of water to a boil, reduce to a simmer and cook the parsnips for 18 to 20 minutes or until soft. Drain, then place in a food processor with the olive oil and roasted garlic flesh. Blend until smooth, then season to taste.

4. Heat a little oil in a large non-stick frying pan over high heat and sear the scallops on each side until they have browned (about 2 minutes each side, depending on size).

5. Spoon the purée onto each plate. Arrange a few scallops on top and garnish with a sprinkling of fresh chives.

TIP Eat lots of scallops for a healthy heart. They're full of vitamin B12 (which keeps homocysteine low and therefore protects against heart attacks and strokes) and magnesium (relaxes blood vessels, thus improving blood flow) and potassium (also keeping blood pressure low).

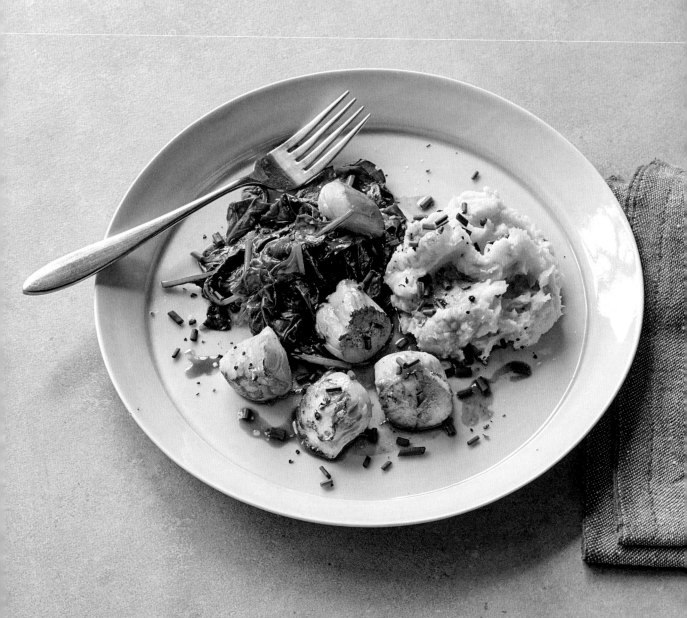

THAI RED CHICKEN CURRY

The Paleo diet is dairy-free but you can use coconut milk for when you're craving something with a lovely creamy texture. However, be aware that coconut milk is high in saturated fat so try to use the "light" version whenever you can.

324 CALORIES | 8G FAT | 2G SATURATES | 5G CARBS | 3.5G SUGAR | 1G SALT | 56G PROTEIN | 3G FIBER

SERVES 4

1 tablespoon olive oil

1 large onion, finely chopped

4 skinless chicken breasts (2 pounds in total), sliced

1-inch piece fresh ginger, grated

1 garlic clove, crushed

2 tablespoons Thai red curry paste

¼ cup plus 2 tablespoons vegetable stock

3½ tablespoons light coconut milk

2 chiles, finely chopped

7 ounces (about 5 cups) fresh spinach

a handful of fresh cilantro, chopped

1. Heat the olive oil in a large, non-stick saucepan and sweat the onion for 3 to 5 minutes, turning constantly.

2. Add the chicken to the pan and cook, stirring, for an additional 5 minutes.

3. Add the ginger, garlic, curry paste, and stock and cook, stirring, for a minute. Then add the coconut milk, reduce the heat to low, cover, and simmer for 12 to 15 minutes.

4. Remove the lid, add the chile and spinach, and cook for an additional 5 minutes, then take off the heat.

5. Divide the curry between four bowls and serve with a sprinkling of fresh cilantro.

TIP As always when buying curry pastes, read the label and check there aren't any preservatives or artificial colors or added flavorings. Brands like Aroy-D and Mae Ploy are Paleo-friendly, or you could always make your own.

CHINESE CHICKEN STIR-FRY

Over the years, I've been very lucky to spend a lot of time in Hong Kong and Shanghai, where I've tasted some of the best Chinese cuisine, with no starch or MSG in sight! In fact, Chinese food, when cooked properly, is very often light and extremely healthy and this stir-fry makes the quickest, easiest, most satisfying weeknight supper.

317 CALORIES | 8G FAT | 1.5G SATURATES | 10G CARBS | 8G SUGAR | 0.4G SALT | 50G PROTEIN | 1.6G FIBER

SERVES 4

1 tablespoon olive oil

4 large skinless chicken breasts, sliced

1 small red onion, sliced

6 to 8 button mushrooms, chopped

1 × 8-ounce can water chestnuts, drained

4 bok choy, leaves separated

1 small red bird's-eye chile, finely chopped

1 teaspoon freshly ground black pepper

1 tablespoon raw unrefined honey

1 tablespoon sesame oil

a handful of fresh chives, finely chopped

1. Heat ½ tablespoon of the olive oil in a large non-stick wok over high heat and stir-fry the chicken until sealed on all sides, then take out of the pan and set aside.

2. Heat the remaining olive oil in the wok, add the onion and mushrooms and stir-fry for 3 to 4 minutes, then add the water chestnuts, bok choy, chile, and pepper, and return the chicken to the pan. Stir-fry over high heat for 2 to 3 minutes, stirring all the time.

3. Take the wok off the heat, add the honey and sesame oil, and stir to coat all the ingredients.

4. Serve immediately with a sprinkling of chopped fresh chives.

TIP Most processed honey today has been heated and filtered which sadly robs it of all its many nutritional benefits and therefore, raw honey is a far superior product. It is generally more solid than regular honey, but if you heat it a little it will melt and can then be drizzled.

FISH STEW
WITH BLACK OLIVES

This dish is incredibly simple to make, but tastes delicious and fills you up with high-quality protein so keeps the hunger pangs at bay. It's both a great dinner party recipe and a brilliant weeknight supper option and the leftovers, steeped in the flavors for longer, are even tastier the following day. Serve with some purple-sprouting broccoli or asparagus if you'd like a few greens on the side.

319 CALORIES | 10G FAT | 1.5G SATURATES | 6G CARBS | 5.5G SUGAR | 2G SALT | 50G PROTEIN | 2.6G FIBER

- -

SERVES 4

1 tablespoon olive oil

1 medium yellow onion, finely chopped

1 × 14.5-ounce can chopped tomatoes

2 garlic cloves, finely chopped

1 cup vegetable stock

1 teaspoon fennel seeds

1 × 6-ounce can pitted black olives, drained

1½ pounds skinless white fish, cut into large chunks

10½ ounces raw peeled king shrimp

a handful of flat-leaf parsley, finely chopped

1. Heat the oil in a large cast-iron casserole pan over high heat and sauté the onions for 2 to 3 minutes.

2. Add the tomatoes and garlic and cook down for a few minutes, then add the stock, fennel seeds, olives, fish, and shrimp, and reduce the heat to low. Cover and cook for 5 minutes until just opaque (so the fish doesn't fall apart).

3. Remove the lid, turn up the heat, and cook for an additional 2 to 3 minutes.

4. Serve immediately with a sprinkling of fresh parsley.

- -

TIP If you like a varied mix of seafood, you could add some clams and mussels and make it to be more like a bouillabaisse (a traditional French seafood soup).

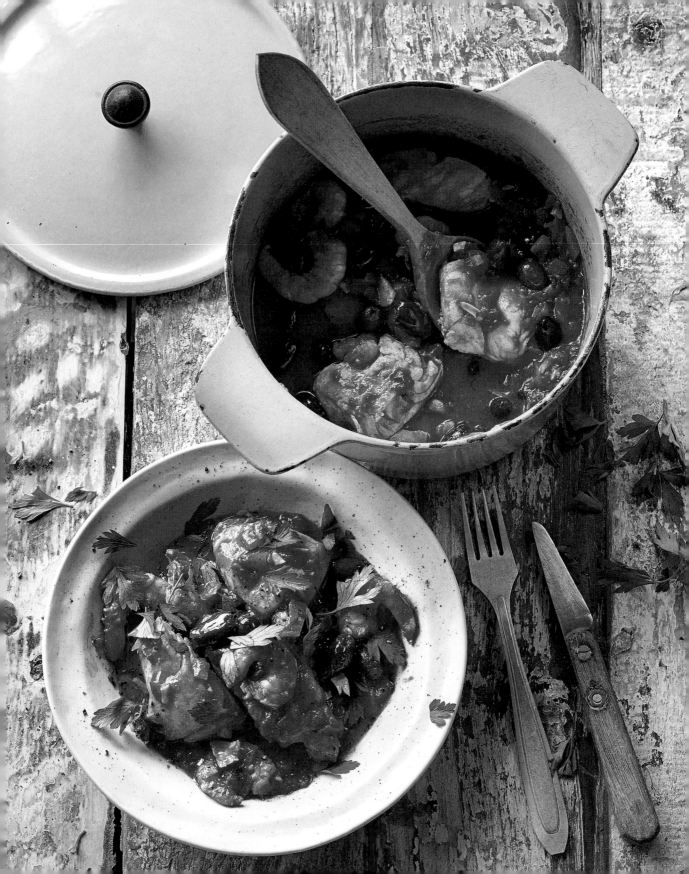

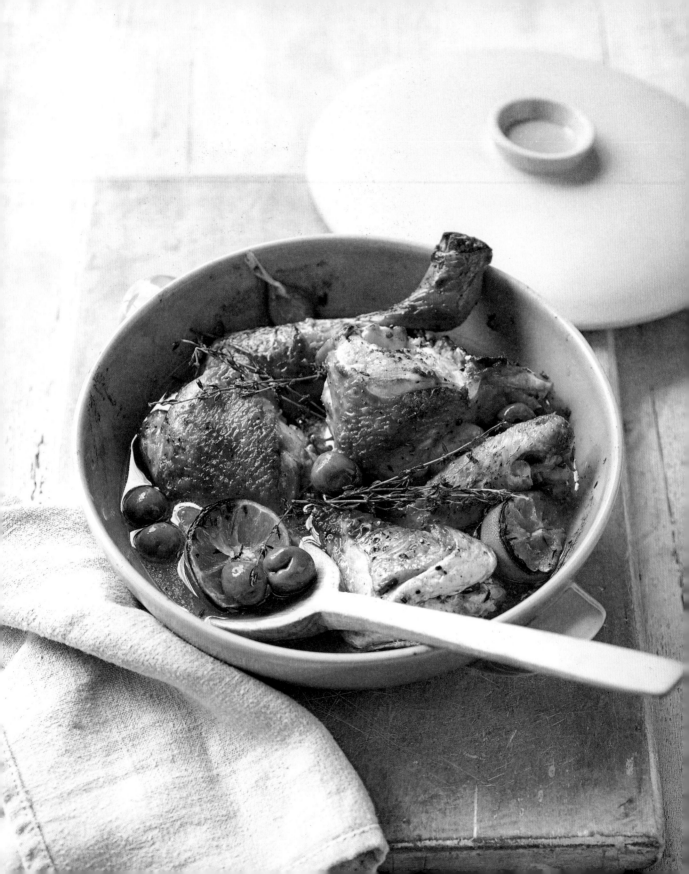

LEMON THYME CHICKEN

This is wonderful over any kind of wilted greens as they absorb all the lovely cooking juices.

555 CALORIES | 19G FAT | 4G SATURATES | 7G CARBS | 7G SUGAR | 2G SALT | 87G PROTEIN | 3G FIBER

SERVES 4

1 tablespoon olive oil

sea salt and freshly ground
   black pepper

1 chicken (approx. 5 pounds),
   cut into 8 pieces

2 lemons, halved

2 tablespoons maple syrup

3 garlic cloves, crushed

1 cup green olives, pitted

2 sprigs of thyme

¾ cup vegetable stock

7 ounces (about 5 cups) fresh
   spinach

1. Add a drizzle of olive oil to a large cast-iron casserole pan and place over high heat. When the oil is hot, lightly season the chicken pieces with salt and pepper, and then sear for about 4 minutes on each side.

2. Squeeze the juice from two of the lemon halves over the chicken and add the squeezed skins to the pan. Add the remaining two lemon halves to the pan together with the maple syrup, garlic, olives, thyme, and stock.

3. Bring to a boil then lower the heat, cover, and simmer for 30 minutes.

4. Serve hot on a bed of spinach or greens of your choice.

TIP Chicken skin has acquired a very bad "high fat" reputation over the years, which is a shame as it turns out that most of the fat is actually healthy, unsaturated fat, and cooking with the skin keeps the chicken flavorful and moist, which reduces the need for extra seasoning.

TANDOORI CHICKEN

This makes a great alternative roast as it's packed full of flavor and is wonderfully simple to prepare.

754 CALORIES | 15G FAT | 5G SATURATES | 1G CARBS | 0.2G SUGAR | 1G SALT | 153G PROTEIN | 0.9G FIBER

- -

SERVES 4

1 large (3½-pound) chicken

1 lemon, quartered

sea salt and freshly ground black pepper

½ cup light coconut milk

1½ teaspoons ground cumin

1½ teaspoons chile powder

1 teaspoon ground turmeric

1 teaspoon ground coriander

1 teaspoon garam masala

4 garlic cloves, crushed

for the salad

7 ounces (about 5 cups) arugula

a handful of fresh cilantro

a handful of fresh mint

1. Preheat the oven to 400°F.

2. Place the chicken in a roasting pan and place the lemon quarters inside the bird. Season lightly with salt and pepper.

3. Place all the remaining ingredients in a bowl and mix together well. Divide this marinade in half and set one half aside.

4. Baste the chicken thoroughly all over with half the marinade and roast in the oven for 45 minutes. Remove the bird from the oven and baste all over again with the remaining marinade, and then roast for an additional 45 minutes or until the thigh juices run clear when tested with a skewer.

5. Serve the chicken with a fresh green herb salad of arugula, cilantro, and mint.

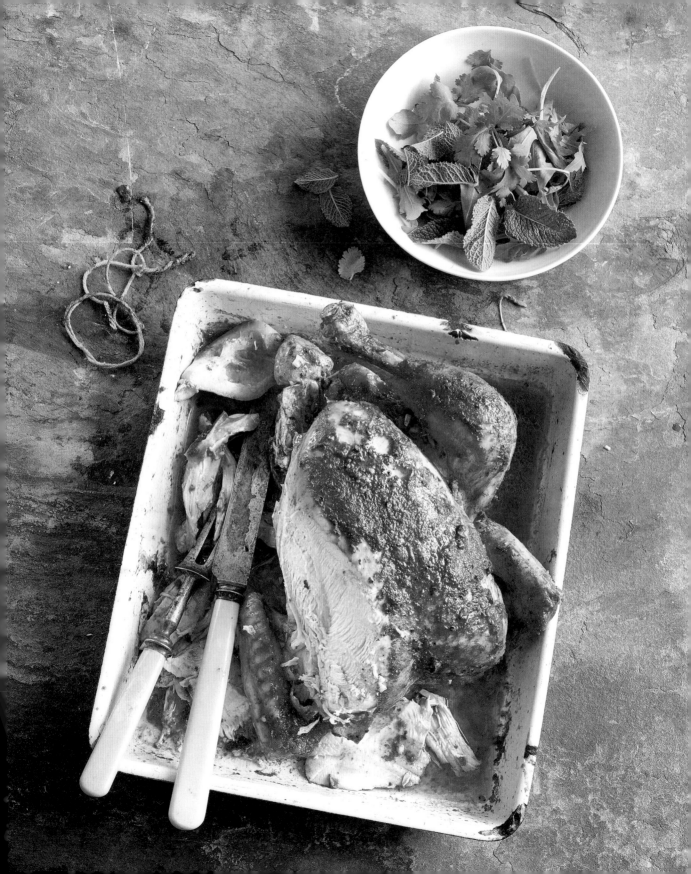

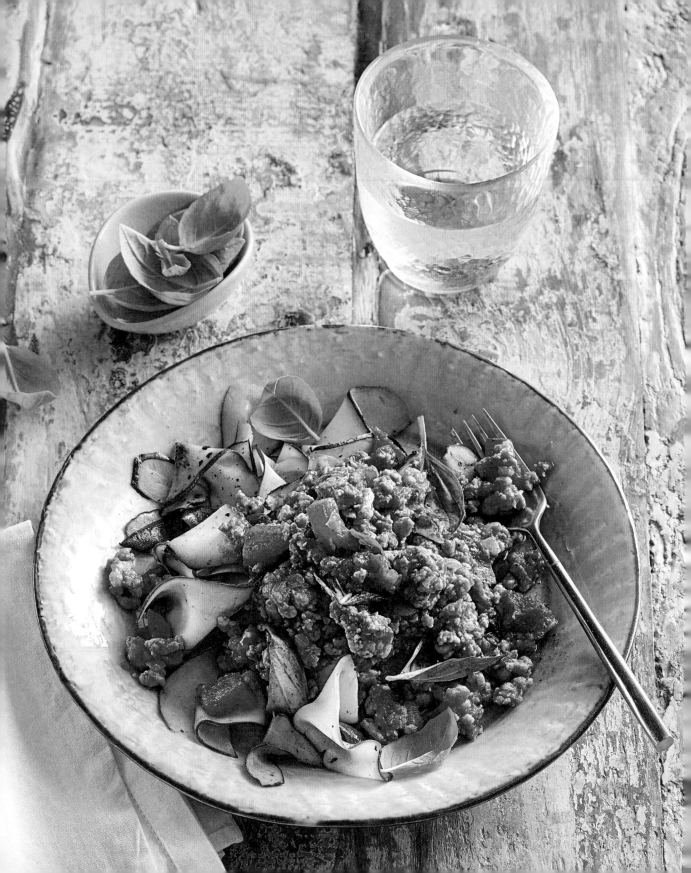

CHICKEN MINCE BOLOGNESE

This is a lovely twist on an old classic. The ground chicken is a delicious alternative to the traditional beef. Plus the sun-dried tomatoes give the dish a wonderfully rich and satisfying flavor, which is of course why we all love spaghetti bolognese in the first place. You can also serve the zucchini noodles with Turkey Meatballs (see next page).

490 CALORIES | 13G FAT | 2.5G SATURATES | 11.5G CARBS | 11G SUGAR | 0.7G SALT | 79G PROTEIN | 4G FIBER

SERVES 4

for the bolognese

1 tablespoon olive oil

1 small yellow onion, finely chopped

2½ pounds lean ground chicken (ask your butcher)

2 garlic cloves

1 × 14.5-ounce can chopped tomatoes

1 tablespoon tomato paste

2 tablespoons chopped sun-dried tomatoes

6 plum tomatoes, chopped

sea salt and freshly ground black pepper

a handful of fresh basil, finely chopped

for the zucchini noodles

1 tablespoon olive oil

2 zucchini, peeled into long ribbons

1. First make the bolognese: Place the olive oil in a large cast-iron pan or non-stick saucepan over high heat and fry the onions, stirring, for 2 to 3 minutes.

2. Add the ground chicken and cook for 2 to 3 minutes, then add the garlic, canned tomatoes, tomato paste, sun-dried tomatoes, and plum tomatoes. Season with salt and pepper, stir to combine, then reduce the heat, cover, and simmer over low heat for 15 minutes.

3. Sprinkle a tablespoon of chopped basil over the pan and stir in well, then cook, uncovered, for a final few minutes.

4. Meanwhile, make the zucchini noodles: In a separate pan, heat the olive oil over medium heat and toss the zucchini ribbons for about 2 to 3 minutes.

5. Divide the zucchini pasta between four serving plates. Add a spoon or two of bolognese, garnish with the remaining basil, and serve straight away.

TIP Zucchini "pasta' is a genius idea and so versatile. In order to make good long spaghetti-like ribbons, it is worth investing in a spiralizer. However, I have also achieved very good results with a simple and more budget-friendly julienne peeler.

TURKEY MEATBALLS

These meatballs are delicious served with a simple salad, or they go very well with zucchini pasta (see previous page).

394 CALORIES | 19G FAT | 2G SATURATES | 10G CARBS | 6G SUGAR | 1.2G SALT | 43G PROTEIN | 5G FIBER

SERVES 4

7 ounces (about 5 cups) mixed salad leaves, to serve

for the meatballs

1 pound ground turkey

1 egg

1 onion, grated

2 to 3 tablespoons homemade or Frank's Hot Wings Sauce (see page 75)

1 teaspoon dried Italian seasoning

1 teaspoon dried parsley

1 teaspoon garlic powder

1 teaspoon onion powder

½ teaspoon sea salt

½ teaspoon black pepper

½ cup almond flour

for the topping

½ cup almond flour

1 teaspoon dried parsley

1 teaspoon crushed black peppercorns

1. Preheat the oven to 400°F and line a baking pan with foil or parchment paper (for easy clean-up). If using foil, spray with a little coconut oil to prevent sticking.

2. Place all the meatball ingredients in a large bowl and use your hands to mix everything together. Divide the mixture into about twenty round balls, then roll them in the topping ingredients to coat lightly and place them on the prepared baking pan.

3. Bake in the oven for 20 to 25 minutes until browned and cooked all the way through.

4. Serve with a simple green salad.

TIP If you prefer a crisp, brown outer crust, fry the meatballs in a sauté pan in 1 tablespoon coconut oil and cook until browned on all sides, then transfer the pan to the oven (or transfer the meatballs to a baking sheet) and bake until firm.

Grating the onion adds moisture to the meatballs. Grate the onion over the bowl in which you are going to mix the meatballs so none of the liquid is lost.

KLEFTIKO

The verb *klevo* in Greek means "to steal" and it's said that when the Greeks were hiding out in the mountains and fighting to liberate themselves from Ottoman rule, they would make this dish in a clay pot and bury it with hot coals under ground until it was done. This way, the cooking smells didn't escape and lead the Ottomans to their hiding places. However, if you don't want to use a clay pot or cook this dish out in your garden, create a parcel for the lamb with parchment paper and foil and this will seal in the heat and cooking juices beautifully.

603 CALORIES | 33G FAT | 13G SATURATES | 0.5G CARBS | 0.5G SUGAR | 0.7G SALT | 76G PROTEIN | 0.6G FIBER

SERVES 4

4.4 pounds leg of lamb on the bone

4 garlic cloves, thinly sliced

sea salt and freshly ground black pepper

1 tablespoon olive oil

juice of 1 lemon

2 tablespoons finely chopped fresh rosemary sprigs

1 whole garlic bulb drizzled in olive oil and wrapped in foil

5 ounces (about 4 cups) mixed salad leaves

a handful of fresh mint

1. Preheat the oven to 425°F.

2. Using a sharp knife, make small incisions all over the leg of lamb and slide garlic slivers into each cut. Season the joint all over with salt and pepper and place in a large roasting pan.

3. Place the oil, lemon juice, and rosemary in a small bowl and stir well together, then rub this marinade all over the lamb joint. Leave for at least 20 minutes for the flavors to infuse.

4. Create a tent for the lamb to cook in by enclosing the pan in a large sheet of baking parchment, covered with a large sheet of foil. Cook in the oven for 20 minutes.

5. Uncover the meat, reduce the heat to 350°F and cook the lamb for 1 hour, then turn the oven off and leave the meat in the hot oven for a final 30 minutes.

6. Serve the lamb with its cooking juices, together with a salad of mixed leaves and fresh mint.

TIP There is nothing like this dish. It's easy to prepare and although it does take a while to cook, this is the reason why it falls off the bone and melts in the mouth.

LAMB SKEWERS

Lamb is a very sturdy meat so you can add heavy flavors to it without overpowering it, unlike fish or white meat. The maple syrup and soy sauce in this recipe go fantastically well with lamb, so make sure the meat is thoroughly coated with the marinade.

446 CALORIES | 23G FAT | 9G SATURATES | 8.5G CARBS | 6G SUGAR | 1.8G SALT | 48G PROTEIN | 3.5G FIBER

SERVES 4

2 garlic cloves, crushed

2 tablespoons coconut aminos

2 teaspoons tomato paste

1 tablespoon maple syrup

a few sprigs of fresh thyme, leaves picked

2 pounds lean boneless lamb, cut into 1 inch cubes

1 medium yellow onion, quartered

1 red pepper, seeded and cut into 1-inch cubes

12 white mushrooms

¾ cup olives

5 ounces (about 4 cups) arugula

1. Preheat the oven to 350°F.

2. Place the garlic, coconut aminos, tomato paste, maple syrup, and thyme in a large bowl and mix together well. Add the lamb and toss in the marinade until thoroughly coated, then cover and place in the refrigerator for 20 minutes.

3. Load each skewer with alternating cubes of lamb, onion, pepper, and mushroom and then place on a foil-lined baking sheet.

4. Place the skewers in the oven and cook for 16 minutes for rare or 20 minutes for medium well-done. Alternatively, broil the skewers, turning and browning all sides until cooked through but still a little pink in the middle.

5. Allow to rest for a minute or two, then serve with a small bowl of olives and a side of fresh arugula.

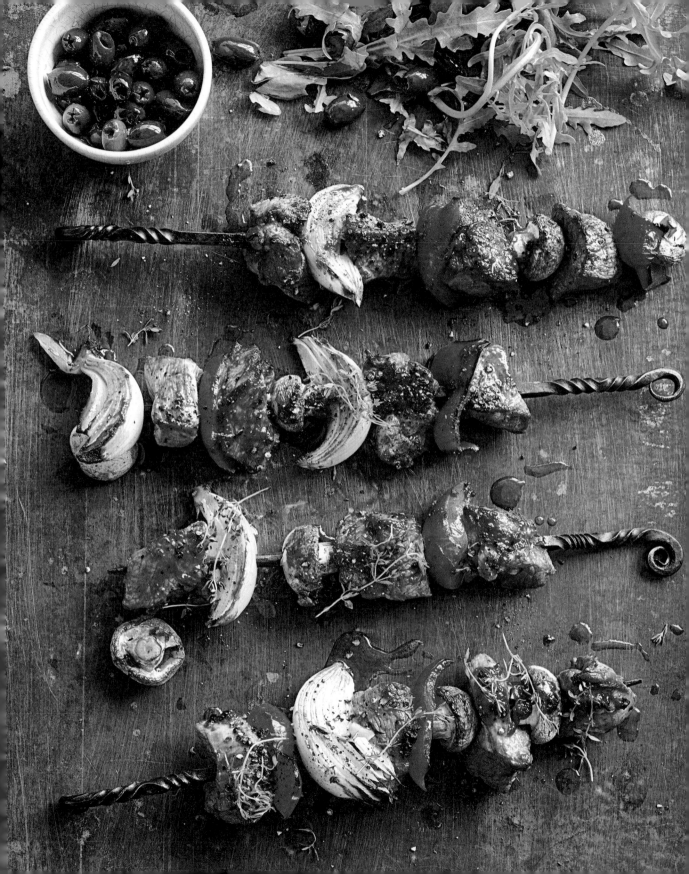

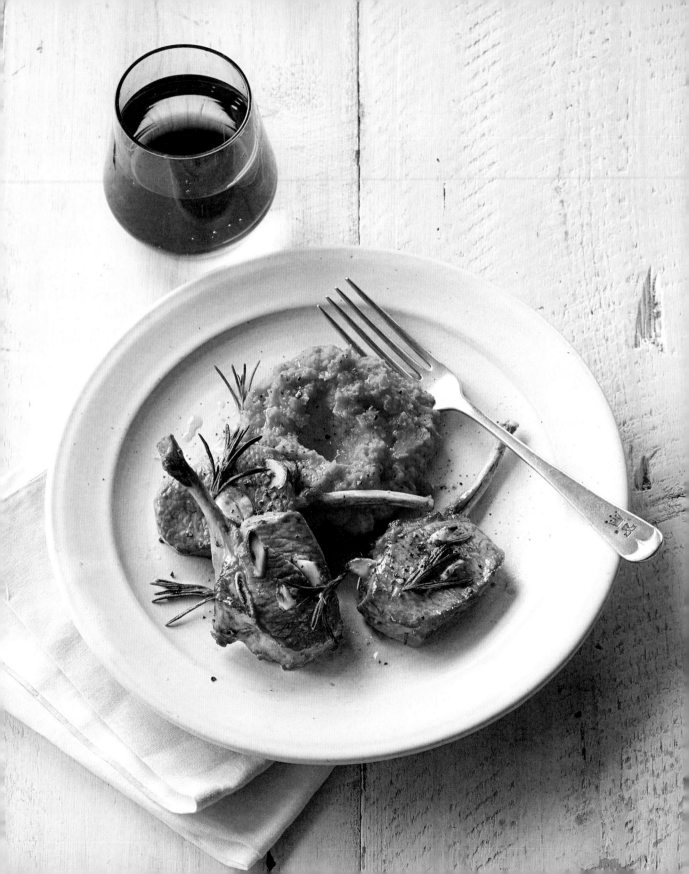

GRILLED LAMB CHOPS ON CARROT PURÉE
WITH ROASTED GARLIC

This is a great midweek supper that only uses a handful of ingredients and is very simple to prepare, yet deliciously satisfying. The carrot purée can be used as a side in many other dishes, such as the Lemon Thyme Chicken on page 129.

486 CALORIES | 26G FAT | 10G SATURATES | 9G CARBS | 8G SUGAR | 0.6G SALT | 51G PROTEIN | 5G FIBER

SERVES 4

1.3 pounds carrots, peeled and roughly chopped

12 lamb chops or cutlets (about 4 ounces each), trimmed of fat

2 garlic cloves, thinly sliced

4 sprigs fresh rosemary, cut into thirds

2 tablespoons olive oil

sea salt and freshly ground black pepper

1. Preheat the oven 350°F.

2. Place the carrots in a saucepan of boiling water and cook for 20 to 25 minutes until soft.

3. Meanwhile, using a sharp knife, cut a few incisions in the lamb and slide in a few garlic slivers and a sprig of rosemary in each chop. Place on a foil-lined baking pan and roast in the oven for 10 to 12 minutes (depending on size).

4. Drain the carrots, transfer to a food processor, and add the olive oil. Season with salt and pepper to taste and process to a smooth purée.

5. Serve the lamb with the carrot purée and garnish with some fresh rosemary.

TIP The beta-carotene that carrots are incredibly rich in can slow down signs of ageing as it acts as an antioxidant and protects against cell damage. It's then converted to vitamin A in the liver and there also assists with flushing toxins out of the body.

BEEF BURGER
IN AN EGGPLANT BUN

You do need a knife and fork to eat this but it has a really nice texture and is a much better alternative to eating the burger on its own.

373 CALORIES | 25G FAT | 9G SATURATES | 7.5G CARBS | 6G SUGAR | 1.7G SALT | 26G PROTEIN | 5G FIBER

- -

SERVES 4

olive oil, for frying

1 eggplant, sliced into 8 rounds

red onion, thinly sliced

1 little gem lettuce or ½ head of romaine

1 tablespoon homemade ketchup (see page 26)

for the burgers

1 pound lean ground beef

1 egg

1 tablespoon Dijon mustard

½ red onion, finely chopped

1 garlic clove, crushed

1 teaspoon salt

½ teaspoon pepper

1 teaspoon onion powder (optional)

½ teaspoon cayenne pepper

1 tablespoon chopped parsley

for the guacamole

1 avocado

juice of 1 lime

a handful of cilantro

1 red or green chile, seeded and finely chopped

1. Place all the burger ingredients in a large bowl and mix together with your hands, then shape into four burgers.

2. Spray a non-stick frying pan with a little olive oil and fry the burgers over medium heat for 3 to 4 minutes on each side or until cooked to your liking. (Alternatively, oven cook them for 20 to 25 minutes in a 400°F oven, but don't forget to flip them halfway through.)

3. Meanwhile, heat a little oil in a second non-stick pan and fry the eggplant slices over medium to high heat for 23 minutes on each side.

4. Place all the guacamole ingredients in a bowl and mash everything together with a fork.

5. Stack each burger on an eggplant slice and layer up with salad, red onion, guacamole, and tomato ketchup, and serve immediately.

- -

TIP When cooking burgers, try to resist flipping too often. It is tempting but they can fall apart if you do.

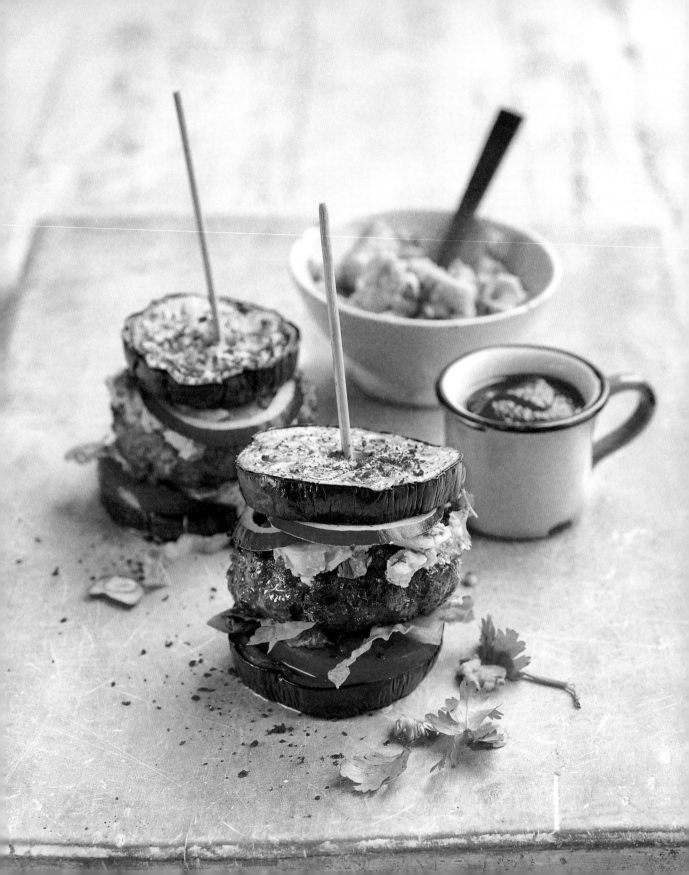

SIRLOIN STEAK

Sirloin is a lovely cut of meat as it has just the right amount of fat to keep it lovely and tender while it cooks, and this is simply the best way to cook it. I recommend you use a barbecue with a lid or a large, smoking-hot grill pan.

927 CALORIES | 36G FAT | 14G SATURATES | 2G CARBS | 2G SUGAR | 1G SALT | 148G PROTEIN | 0.8G FIBER

- -

SERVES 4 TO 6

4 to 6 pounds sirloin beef

2 teaspoons olive oil

sea salt and freshly ground black pepper

canned hearts of palm, sliced

7 ounces (about 5 cups) green salad, including arugula balsamic vinaigrette (see page 98)

1. Place a grill pan over high heat and let it heat up.

2. Rub the steak all over with a little oil and season with salt and pepper.

3. Sear the steak on the grill pan for about 2 to 3 minutes, then turn and sear again for another 2 to 3 minutes. Repeat this until the beef has rotated fully and is seared on all sides, then rest for 15 minutes. (If you are using an outdoor grill with a lid, ensure it is closed while the meat rests.)

4. Transfer the meat to a board and rest for a few additional minutes, then slice into large steaks.

5. Serve with sliced hearts of palm and some fresh green salad, drizzled with a little balsamic vinaigrette.

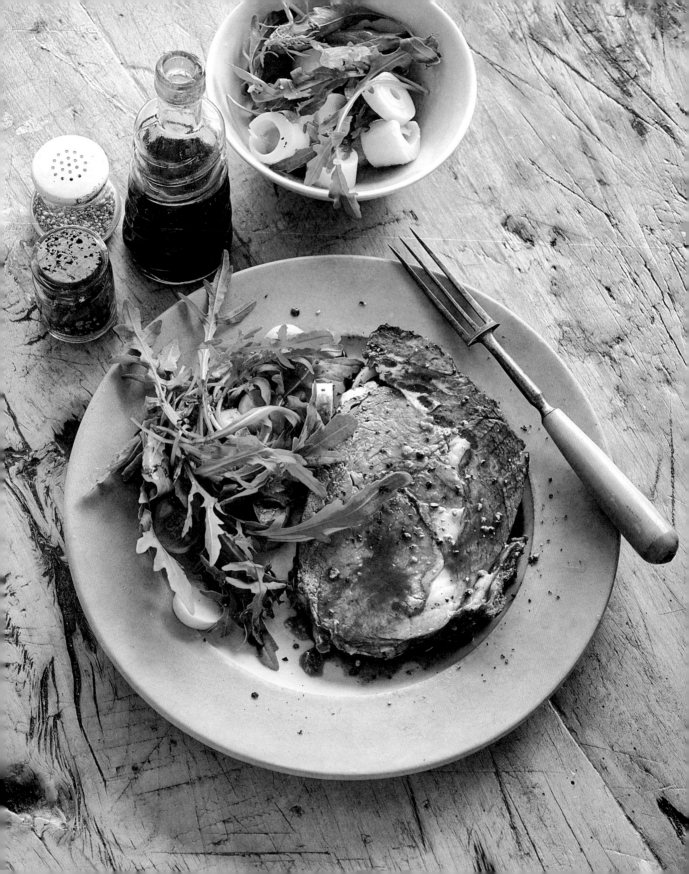

FILET MIGNON
WITH CARAMELIZED ONIONS

A good filet mignon should be so tender you can cut it with a fork. It's often a very expensive choice on a restaurant menu and so it's much better to make it at home. I recommend you source it from your local butcher and don't overcook it, and also don't forget to take the steaks out of the fridge 1 to 2 hours prior to cooking, to bring them up to room temperature. This helps the meat brown nicely as you don't waste heat from the pan taking the chill off its surface area.

760 CALORIES | 46G FAT | 10G SATURATES | 18G CARBS | 15G SUGAR | 0.3G SALT | 46G PROTEIN | 7G FIBER

SERVES 2

2 × 7-ounce filet mignon steaks

3 tablespoons extra virgin olive oil

sea salt and freshly ground black pepper

8 ounces fresh mushrooms (any variety), chopped

1 tablespoon chopped fresh thyme

¾ cup red wine

5½ ounces carrots

for the caramelized onions

3 onions, thinly sliced

2 tablespoons extra virgin olive oil, plus more as needed

sea salt and freshly ground black pepper, to taste

1. First make the caramelized onions: Place the onions in a large frying pan over medium-high heat, cover and cook, stirring infrequently, until they are dry and almost sticking to the pan (about 20 minutes).

2. Stir in the oil and a large pinch of salt, then reduce the heat to medium-low and cook, stirring occasionally and adding oil as needed to keep them from sticking without getting greasy, for 40 to 60 minutes, depending on how silky you want them. Season to taste and set aside.

3. Meanwhile, brush the steaks all over with a little olive oil and season lightly with salt and pepper. Place a large grill pan over medium high heat and, when hot, add the steaks and cook for 2 to 3 minutes on each side (or until done to your liking), then remove from the pan and set aside.

4. Add the remaining olive oil to the pan, add the mushrooms, and cook over high heat for 5 to 10 minutes until golden brown.

5. Add the wine and thyme to the pan, bring to a simmer, and cook for 3 to 4 minutes until the wine has reduced slightly.

6. Plate the steaks with a spoonful of sauce, the caramelized onions on the side, and a few carrots too, if you like.

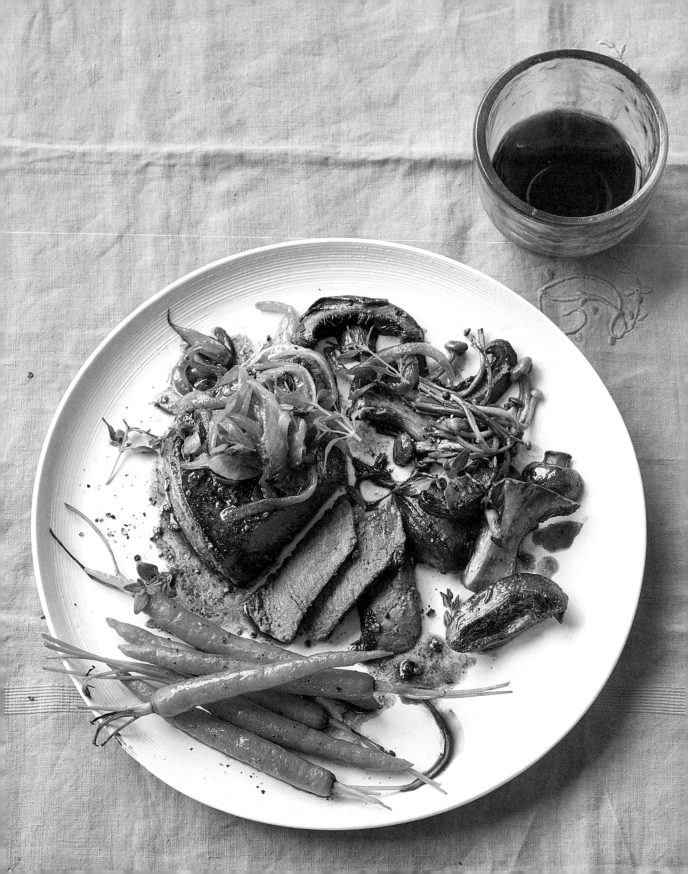

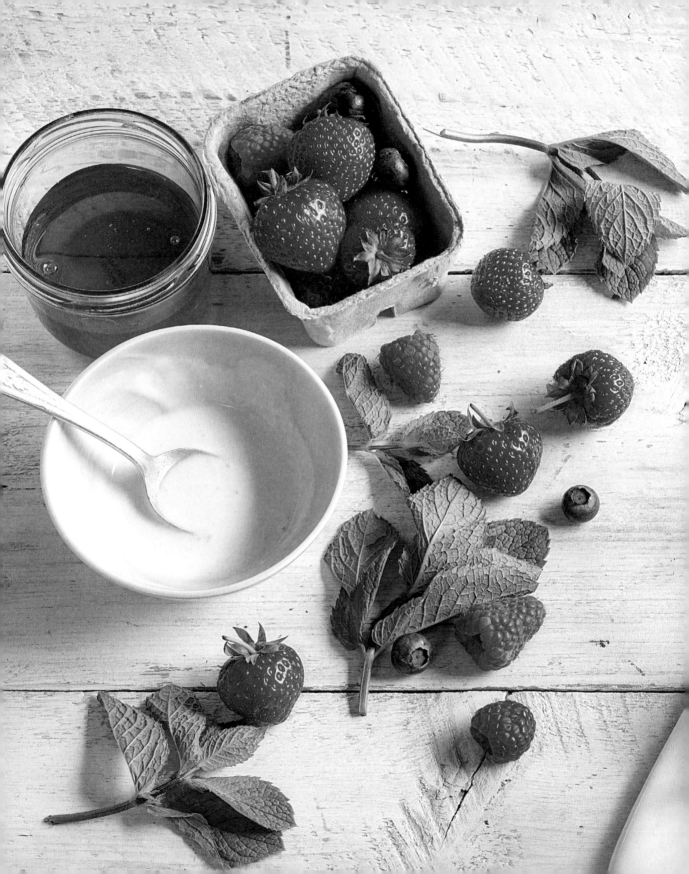

DESSERTS

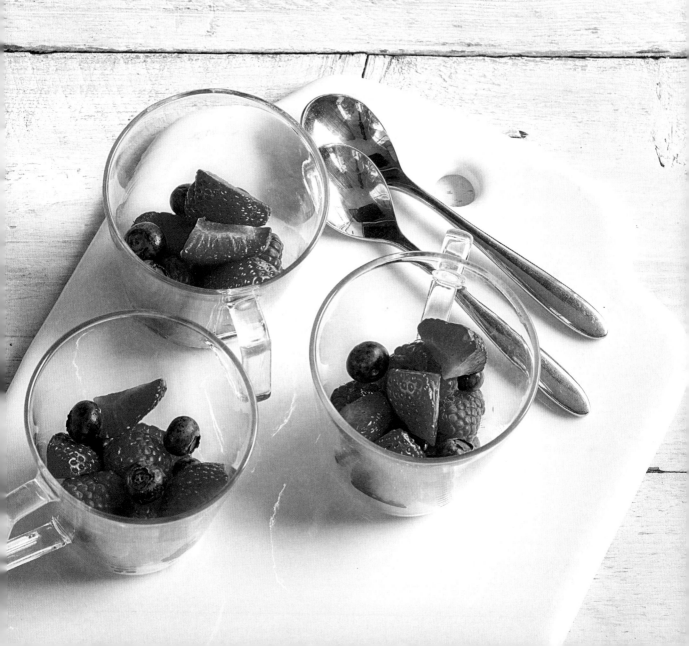

APPLE PIE

I try to avoid desserts as a rule, but of course there are always those days when one savory course just isn't enough and what you really want is something sweet. This apple pie is still Paleo and will hopefully hit the spot.

442 CALORIES | 21G FAT | 1.7G SATURATES | 49G CARBS | 42G SUGAR | 0.1G SALT | 12G PROTEIN | 6G FIBER

- -

SERVES 4

5 Granny Smith apples, peeled, cored and sliced

½ teaspoon cinnamon

juice of 2 oranges

3 tablespoons maple syrup

for the topping

3 tablespoons maple syrup

1½ cups almond flour or coconut flour

3 egg whites, whisked

1. Preheat the oven to 350°F.

2. Place the apples, cinnamon, orange juice, and maple syrup in a large bowl and mix together until the apple pieces are thoroughly coated. Tip the fruit into a baking dish and bake for 35 minutes.

3. Meanwhile, place all the topping ingredients in a bowl and mix together thoroughly.

4. When the apple is cooked, spread the topping mix evenly over the top, then return to the oven and bake for an additional 30 minutes. Serve slightly warm.

- -

TIP Any leftovers will also make a very tasty breakfast.

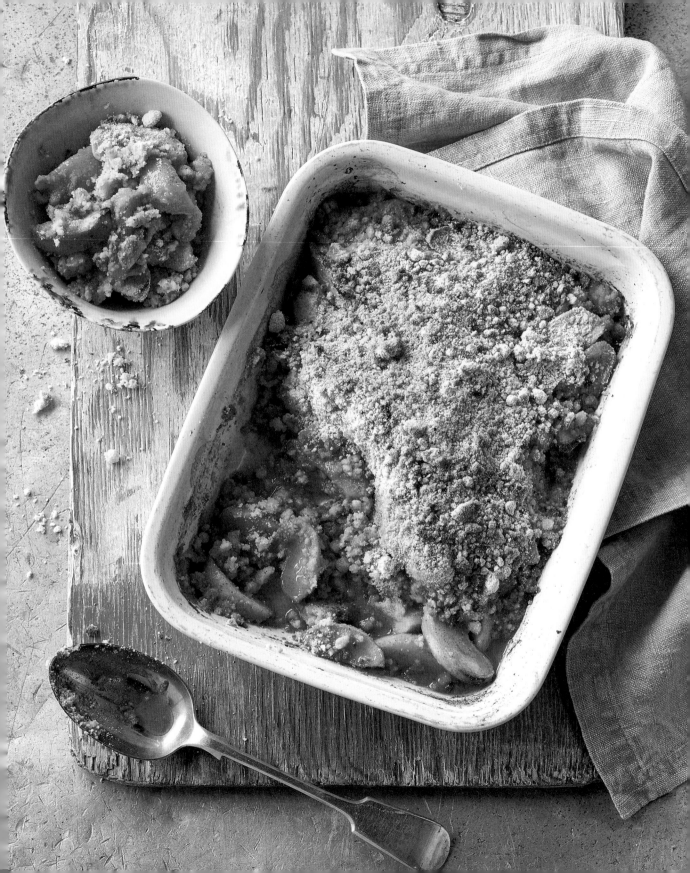

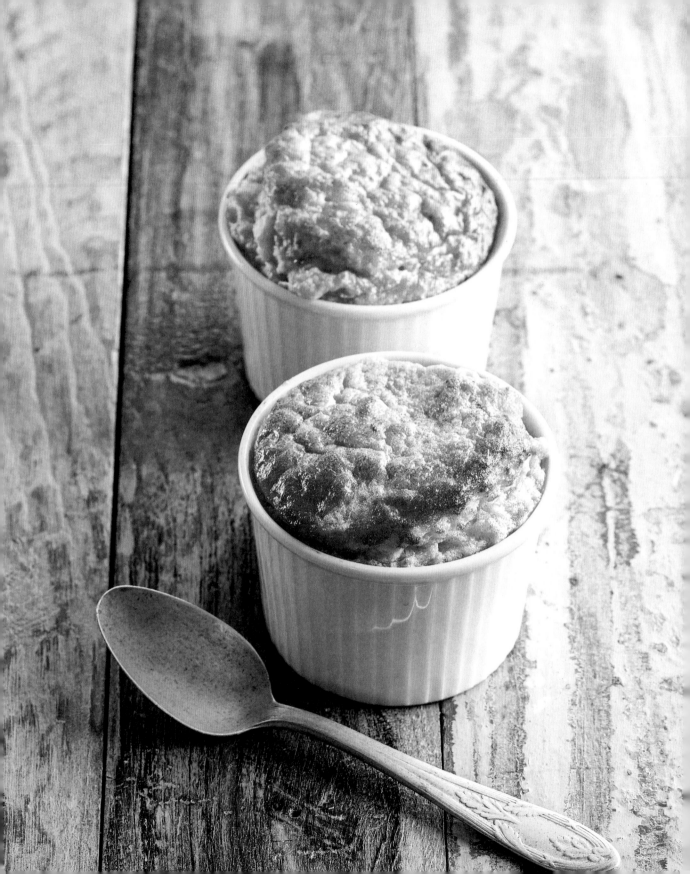

BANANA SOUFFLÉ

The more you whisk the eggs, the higher the soufflés rise in the oven...

189 CALORIES | 8G FAT | 2.5G SATURATES | 16G CARBS | 14G SUGAR | 0.4G SALT | 12G PROTEIN | 0.7G FIBER

SERVES 4 TO 6

2 ripe bananas

1 teaspoon vanilla paste
 (or extract)

2 tablespoons maple syrup
 (at room temp)

6 eggs

1. Preheat the oven to 400°F.

2. Mash the bananas with the vanilla in a bowl, then add the maple syrup and mix well.

3. Separate the eggs and, using an electric mixer, whisk the egg whites until they form soft peaks. Add the yolks to the banana mixture and stir well. Gently fold the two mixtures together and divide between four to six silicone ramekins (if not using silicone, oil very lightly).

4. Bake in the oven for 15 minutes until well risen. Serve immediately.

TIP Make sure you whisk your eggs in a very clean mixing bowl. Before using, I always rinse mine with boiling water and dry with a clean tea towel to ensure it's completely free from grease.

COCONUT EGG CUSTARD

This is a very light dessert. The custard should have a lovely silky smooth texture and the trick to achieving this is to cook it for a long time over a very low heat.

234 CALORIES | 15G FAT | 6G SATURATES | 9G CARBS | 7.5G SUGAR | 0.5G SALT | 16G PROTEIN | 0.8G FIBER

SERVES 4

8 eggs

1 cup plus 2 tablespoons light
   coconut milk

1 teaspoon ground cinnamon

2 tablespoons maple syrup

4 kumquats

1. Crack the eggs into a large bowl and whisk together. Add the coconut milk, cinnamon, and maple syrup and whisk to combine, then divide between four ramekin dishes.

2. Bring a saucepan of water to a boil, and place the ramekins in a steamer on top of the pan. Turn the heat down as low as you can and simmer for 18 to 20 minutes.

3. Serve with fresh kumquats or fruit of your choice.

TIP Cinnamon is loaded with antioxidants, more than any other spice (even super-spices like garlic and oregano), plus it helps the body fight infections and repairs tissue damage.

BANANA FRITTERS

This is the perfect, easy dish to rustle up in minutes when you really need something for that sweet tooth.

658 CALORIES | 39G FAT | 17G SATURATES | 47G CARBS | 21G SUGAR | 0.3G SALT | 19G PROTEIN | 15G FIBER

SERVES 4

4 ripe bananas

2 eggs

1½ cups almond flour

coconut oil, for frying

1¼ cups coconut flour

1. Place the bananas in a large bowl and, with a fork, mash until smooth. Add the eggs and almond flour and whisk until combined.

2. Heat a little coconut oil in a large non-stick frying pan over medium heat. When hot, drop small spoonfuls of banana batter into the oil and press down flat.

3. Sprinkle with a little coconut flour and fry for a few minutes, then flip the fritter over with a spatula and cook on the other side. Repeat until all the batter is used up. Serve warm.

TIP Bananas are very interesting in relation to their carbohydrate and sugar content. They are very sweet, especially when ripe and they do contain 14 to 15 grams of sugar, yet they have a low-GI value, which means the sugar doesn't result in a short, fast energy spike. This is largely down to their high fiber content as this helps regulate digestion (i.e. the conversion of carbs to simple sugars), and in particular to a type of fiber called pectin, as this moderates the impact of banana consumption on our blood sugar and supports our overall digestive health.

COCONUT BERRIES

This is a delicious, light dessert—perfect for summer when so many berries are in season. Obviously the coconut milk does have a high fat content, so use sparingly if you are trying to keep the weight off or save this up for the weekend. You could also try this with light coconut milk, but you don't get quite as much of the thick creamy part as you need so it's not as tasty.

141 CALORIES | 9G FAT | 8G SATURATES | 11G CARBS | 10G SUGAR | 0G SALT | 2G PROTEIN | 3G FIBER

SERVES 4

1 × 14-ounce can coconut milk

1 tablespoon raw honey (at room temperature)

1 teaspoon vanilla extract

1 pound (about 3 cups) mixed berries

mint, for garnish

1. Open the can of coconut milk and remove the thick creamy part on top, reserving the thinner milk for use in a smoothie (see pages 39 to 43). Keeping the can in the fridge for a few hours will help the milk separate.

2. Place the coconut cream in a bowl and, using an electric whisk, fluff it up into soft peaks. Add the honey and vanilla and whisk a little more.

3. Place a few berries into the bottom of four glasses and top with a layer of coconut cream, then repeat both these steps until you reach the top. Garnish with a sprig of mint and serve immediately.

TIP Because of their fiber and moisture content, berries give you a nice sense of fullness, which means they round off a meal very nicely. They're also chock-full of antioxidants.

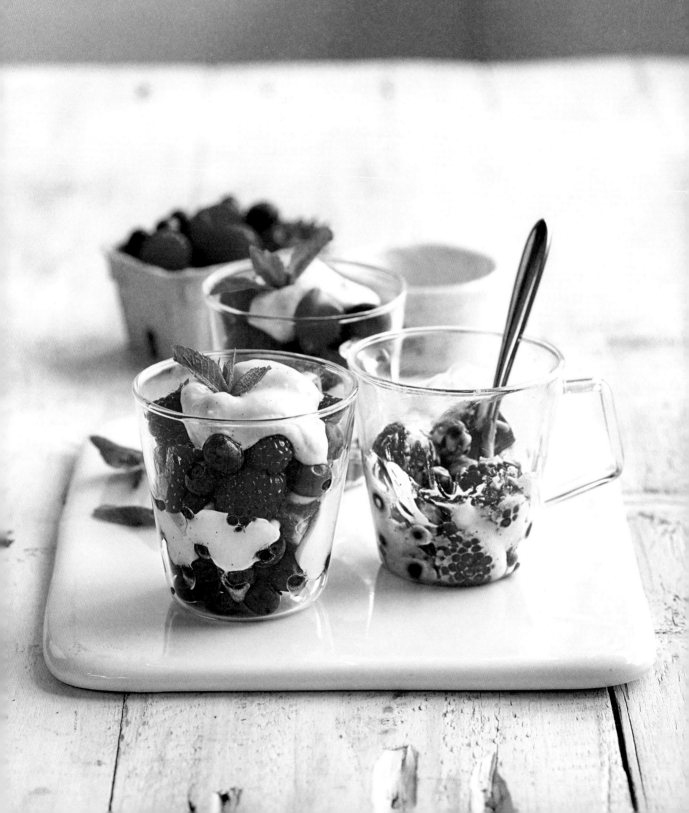

INDEX

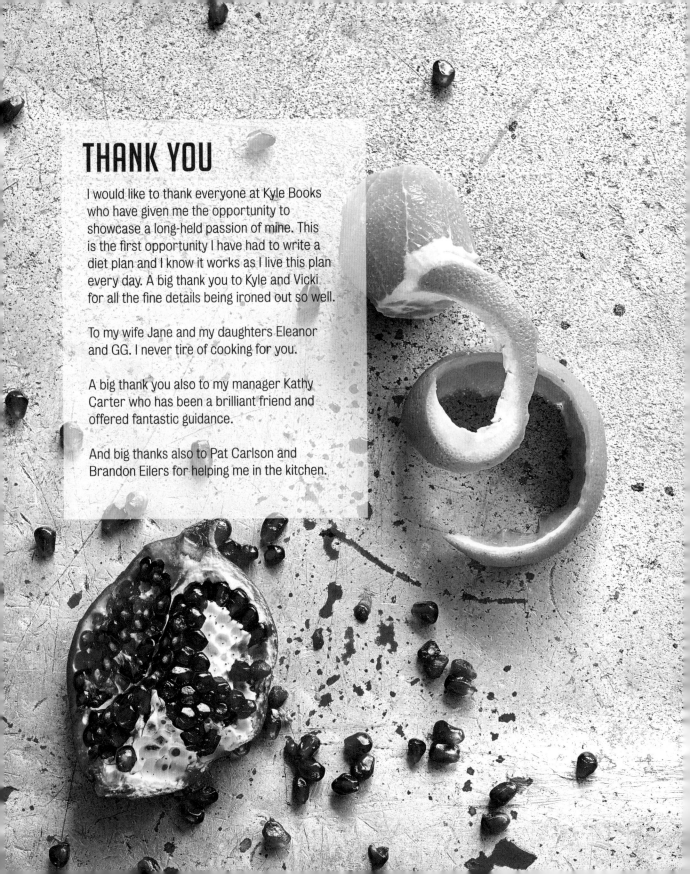

THANK YOU

I would like to thank everyone at Kyle Books who have given me the opportunity to showcase a long-held passion of mine. This is the first opportunity I have had to write a diet plan and I know it works as I live this plan every day. A big thank you to Kyle and Vicki for all the fine details being ironed out so well.

To my wife Jane and my daughters Eleanor and GG. I never tire of cooking for you.

A big thank you also to my manager Kathy Carter who has been a brilliant friend and offered fantastic guidance.

And big thanks also to Pat Carlson and Brandon Eilers for helping me in the kitchen.